Museum-based Art Therapy

T0199832

This practical and inspirational resource offers a wide range of information about museum-based art therapy and wellness programming in various museums.

Featuring contributions from art therapists and access professionals from various museum-based wellness programs, the book describes museum-based art therapy, education, access, and inclusion to enlarge the scope of professional development and higher education training in art therapy and its relation to museum studies. Chapter examples of successful museum art therapy and wellness initiatives increase awareness about the role of art therapy in museums and the role of museums in building healthy societies and improving lives. The text also contributes to the field of art therapy by deconstructing traditional narratives about therapy being conceived only as a clinical treatment, and by introducing arts-based approaches and strategies in museums as expanding territories for being proactive in community health and wellness.

Museum-based Art Therapy is a valuable guide for art students who are interested in working in museum education, access and disabilities, or museum studies, and graduates and professionals working across the disciplines of museums, art therapy, and disability studies.

Mitra Reyhani Ghadim, **DAT, ATR-BC, LCAT**, is an art therapist, author, and educator. She worked as a museum art therapist for nearly a decade, creating several art therapy programs for various populations.

Lauren Daugherty, **LMHC, ATR-P**, is an art therapist at the Eskenazi Museum of Art at Indiana University Bloomington where she established the first museum art therapy program at a university museum in the U.S.

"This richly diverse text documents the exciting partnership that museums and community-based art therapy are creating at the intersection of inclusivity, accessibility, wellness, and education. At its center is the shifting power of museums to provide restorative spaces of reparation and reimagination. A wealth of information details the formation of effective programs and models, strategies for collaboration, critical reflection, and engaging activities and processes. This text will be celebrated as an invaluable guide for multiplying museum-based arts and wellness programs that strengthen communities."

—**Lynn Kapitan, PhD, ATR-BC, HLM**, *is founder, professor, and director of the Professional Doctor of Art Therapy program at Mount Mary University*

Museum-based Art Therapy

A Collaborative Effort with Access, Education, and Public Programs

**Edited by Mitra Reyhani Ghadim
and Lauren Daugherty**

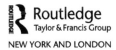
Routledge
Taylor & Francis Group

NEW YORK AND LONDON

First published 2022
by Routledge
605 Third Avenue, New York, NY 10158

and by Routledge
2 Park Square, Milton Park, Abingdon, Oxon, OX14 4RN

Routledge is an imprint of the Taylor & Francis Group, an informa business

© 2022 Taylor & Francis

The right of Mitra Reyhani Ghadim and Lauren Daugherty to be identified as the authors of the editorial material, and of the authors for their individual chapters, has been asserted in accordance with sections 77 and 78 of the Copyright, Designs and Patents Act 1988.

Trademark notice: Product or corporate names may be trademarks or registered trademarks, and are used only for identification and explanation without intent to infringe.

Library of Congress Cataloging-in-Publication Data
Names: Ghadim, Mitra Reyhani, editor. | Daugherty, Lauren, editor.
Title: Museum-based art therapy : a collaborative effort with access, education, and public programs / edited by Mitra Reyhani Ghadim and Lauren Daugherty.
Description: New York, NY : Routledge, 2022. | Includes bibliographical references and index.
Identifiers: LCCN 2021022268 (print) | LCCN 2021022269 (ebook) | ISBN 9780367856540 (hardback) | ISBN 9780367856533 (paperback) | ISBN 9781003014386 (ebook)
Subjects: LCSH: Art therapy. | Museums—Therapeutic use.
Classification: LCC RC489.A7 M87 2022 (print) | LCC RC489.A7 (ebook) | DDC 616.89/1656—dc23
LC record available at https://lccn.loc.gov/2021022268
LC ebook record available at https://lccn.loc.gov/2021022269

ISBN: 978-0-367-85654-0 (hbk)
ISBN: 978-0-367-85653-3 (pbk)
ISBN: 978-1-003-01438-6 (ebk)

DOI: 10.4324/9781003014386

Typeset in Times New Roman
by Apex CoVantage, LLC

Contents

vi   *Contents*

Figures

Tables

Contributors

Editor Bios

Dr. Mitra Reyhani Ghadim, LCAT, ATR-BC, is a NYS licensed, registered art therapist, researcher, author, and educator. She works with the NYS Office of Mental Health, currently at Sagamore Children's Psychiatric Center. She worked as a full-time museum art therapist for nearly a decade, making contributions to the Art*Access* Programs and Autism Initiatives of the Queens Museum, as well as Nassau County Museum of the Arts. She also worked in adult clinical settings such as Mount Sinai South Nassau inpatient behavioral unit, in community-based programs for older adults, and is an artist in residence at The Living Museum. She has years of experience working with individuals with mental illness and children and adults with disabilities in museums, community, and clinical settings. She currently teaches at Hofstra University and LIU Post. Mitra holds an M.A. in Creative Arts Therapy, an M.F.A. in Visual Arts, and a doctorate in Art Therapy.

Lauren Daugherty, LMHC, ATR-P, is the Arts-based Wellness Experiences Manger and full-time art therapist at the Sidney and Lois Eskenazi Museum of Art at Indiana University Bloomington. In this inaugural position at the museum, she established art therapy programming for individuals of all ages and abilities, including children from backgrounds of abuse and neglect, individuals with cognitive and developmental disabilities, and Indiana University students. She obtained her master's degree in art therapy from the Herron School of Art and Design at IUPUI where she completed her thesis research on art therapy in art museums. She is passionate about assisting others in personal growth through connecting and responding to museum collections in meaningful ways and utilizing art-making and the creative process to promote health and well-being.

Contributor Bios

Carolyn Brown Treadon, ATR-BC, ATCS, is a Registered and Board Certified art therapist and an Art Therapy Certified Supervisor. She is the Graduate

Program Director for Art Therapy at Edinboro University of Pennsylvania. She received a Bachelor of Science in Psychology and Fine Art from Ohio University, Master of Arts in Expressive Therapy from The University of Louisville and a Ph.D. from Florida State University. She has provided art therapy services in alternative schools and out-patient settings before becoming clinical supervisor of a community based mental health clinic. Carolyn's research includes utilizing art museums in the therapeutic process and using the art therapy process to alter individual's perceptions and attitudes toward individuals with disabilities. She continues to explore how using resources such as the museum and other experience-based practices can further students' knowledge acquisition during their training to become art therapists.

Ashley Hartman, Ph.D., LCAT, LPC, ATR-BC, is an Assistant Professor of Art Therapy at Marywood University. She is an educator, registered art therapist, researcher, and artist. She earned her Doctorate with a specialization in art therapy from Florida State University. Ashley has also worked as an Adjunct Instructor at Florida State University and has worked in diverse community based and clinical settings. She is a licensed creative arts therapist (LCAT) in the state of NY, a licensed professional counselor (LPC), and a board credentialed art therapist (ATR-BC). Ashley's scholarly endeavors focus on the areas of museum-based art therapy, art therapy and intersectional aspects of identity, art therapy with individuals on the Spectrum, and the integration of Eastern philosophical practices in connection to perception of control, anxiety, and mindfulness.

Kathy Dumlao is the Director of Education and Interpretation at the Memphis Brooks Museum of Art. She has served in several roles at the museum over the last 21 years, including in her current role as head of the education department since 2013. In addition to managing both the education and visitor services departments, Kathy oversees the museum's Art Therapy Access Program, manages adult programming, and serves as a member of the museum leadership team. Additionally, Kathy has served on the board of the Tennessee Art Education Association (TAEA) since 2009, including six years as President-elect, President, and Past President. She was awarded the TAEA's Museum Educator of the Year in 2009 and completed the National Art Education Association's School for Art Leaders in 2017. Kathy received her M.A. in Art History from the University of Memphis.

Paige Scheinberg, MS, ATR-BC, RYT, founded SHINE ON Consulting in 2015 with the goal of making well-being and healing more accessible to those in need through creative experiences, integrative approaches, and community partnerships. Paige offers integrative art therapy services, clinical supervision, workshops, and trainings for personal and professional development, which incorporate creativity, mindfulness, and positive psychology theory, approaches, and practices. Currently, she primarily works with cancer survivors and caregivers in an adult oncology outpatient clinic, as well as offers museum-based art therapy offerings at the Brooks Museum. Paige also loves creating and exploring mandalas and enjoys building an international mandala community with her Creating Mandalas team.

Additionally, Paige is committed to raising awareness of and advocating for mental health and art therapy, as well as supporting and empowering fellow advocates. As the TATA Governmental Affairs Co-Chair, Paige co-led the efforts to create a state art therapy license in TN.

Michelle López Torres, ATR, is the National Director of Parent Education Programs at Literacy Partners, leading a family engagement program that centers the voices and experiences of Latinx caregivers as the most powerful influence on a child's early development. She served as Director of Education and Community Engagement at the Children's Museum of Arts and Manager of Art*Access* and Autism Initiatives at Queens Museum, both in New York City. The model Michelle developed for arts programming in community spaces has disseminated through a guide called Room to Grow. She designed emPOWER Parents: Fostering Cross-Cultural Networks between Families Affected by Autism in Queens and Madrid. Michelle has a master's in Creative Arts Therapy from Hofstra University and a bachelor's in Communication Arts from Fordham University. She is an adjunct professor at CUNY's City College's Masters program for Arts & Theater Education.

Vida Sabbaghi is a cultural producer and leader on matters of equity, inclusion, and social justice, is Founder and Executive Director of COPE NYC (Creative Opportunities Promoting Equality) whose mission is to bridge communities through art and design. COPE NYC promotes social relations for all ages and abilities through community art projects, workshops, fashion shows, art exhibits, conferences, and international residencies. Under COPE NYC, Vida partners with cultural institutions to create innovative projects. She works with kindergarten to graduate art students. She also writes articles for art publications. She and Dr. Alice J. Wexler co-edited *Bridging Communities Through Socially Engaged Art*. She received the NYCATA Art Advocate of the Year Award, and the USSEA, Edwin Ziegfeld Service Award for organizing an international conference at Queens Museum. Vida is the Art Director of 630 Flushing Avenue, in Brooklyn, where, under COPE NYC, she mounts rotating exhibitions and runs residencies for Pratt and SVA.

Sarah Pousty is a New York State Licensed Creative Arts Therapist (LCAT) and Registered, Board Certified Art Therapist (ATR-BC) with expertise in clinical practice and community-based approaches. She has provided therapeutic services as part of a milieu for survivors of domestic violence, treatment for young children as part of an outpatient mental health clinic, and developed a community-based visitation program for families navigating the NYC child welfare system, which she now supervises. Sarah wrote a chapter that was included in the anthology titled, *Art Therapy Practices for Resilient Youth: A Strengths-Based Approach to At-Promise Children and Adolescents.*

Alice Garfield has served as the coordinator for MFA Restorative Arts at the Museum of Fine Arts, Boston since 2017, overseeing Artful Healing, Restorative Arts, and Beyond the Spectrum programming. Through these programs, the MFA provides art education and art-making activities to a variety of audiences with a focus on health, wellbeing, accessibility, and inclusion. Alice holds a Masters degree in Art Education from Tufts/SMFA and a Bachelors degree from Pomona College, and is a licensed visual art teacher. She has taught art to students of all ages, interests, and abilities, and passionately pursues facilitating positive growth and change through the arts. Alice is involved in promoting the growing field of arts in health through organizations including the National Organization for Arts in Health (NOAH), AAM, and the Boston Arts Consortium for Health (BACH).

Rachel Shipps is currently an art mentor at Tierra del Sol Foundation, providing direct support to artists with disabilities in their studio practices and their ongoing education in the arts. She held the role of Education Coordinator at the San Francisco Museum of Craft and Design and of Art*Access* Coordinator at the Queens Museum, and is passionate about possibilities for accessibility and collaboration in cultural institutions. Rachel has a B.A. in Psychology and an M.A. in Public Humanities with professional experience in ABA-based instruction, behavior therapy, and non-directive therapeutic play.

Stephen Legari holds a Masters in creative arts therapies from Concordia University and a Masters in couple and family therapy from McGill University. He has worked extensively with individuals, groups, couples, and families in both clinical and non-clinical settings. Since 2017, Stephen has been program officer for art therapy at the Montreal Museum of Fine Arts where he has developed specialized therapy programs for groups, supervised Masters level students, and contributed to numerous publications on the arts in health.

Chloe Hayward is an art therapist, artist, and educator living and working in New York City. She believes in the power of art to heal and has written articles on the subject for Studio Magazine, Pratt Institute, and Artsy Magazine. Chloe serves on the board of directors for Artistic Noise, an organization which provides self-expression through the arts for youth impacted by the justice system. As Associate Director of Education at The Studio Museum in Harlem, she co-creates with her department to provide a robust focus on the intersection between art, education, and mental health, overseeing programs and projects rooted in community care and abolition. Her work uses the power of the creative arts process to heal, bring awareness, and promote social change, equity, and inclusion.

Marie Clapot is Associate Museum Educator for Accessibility at The Metropolitan Museum of Art. In this capacity, she and her colleagues provide oversight of key Access programs while also focusing on embedding accessible and inclusive practices into the fabric of the museum at large. Marie has trained museum professionals in the US and abroad, and consults for nonprofit agencies on accessibility and inclusive practices. She also co-convened the last two Multimodal Approaches to Learning conferences with the Met (2009, 2012). Marie's publications include "Insights from an educator into crafting scent-based experiences in museum galleries" in *Bridging Communities Through Socially Engaged Art*, amongst others. Her research includes the role of olfaction in gallery teaching and learning. She holds a Masters in Art Education from Indiana University, and an MA in Heritage Development from Université de Bretagne Occidentale (UBO), Quimper (France), and an MA in Heritage Development from UBO (Brest).

Preface

Mitra Reyhani Ghadim and Lauren Daugherty

Museums are increasingly becoming interested in utilizing their collections to promote health and well-being in the communities they serve. Some museums have hired art therapists trained in psychological theories and use of art materials, and with deep knowledge and interest in the visual arts, to provide wellness and art therapy programming for their audiences. Other museums have chosen to utilize existing museum educators within their institutions to develop wellness programs. This book illustrates the healing power of the visual arts and, more specifically, provides museum-based art therapists and museum educators examples of select art therapy and wellness-based programs from the United States and Canada, while also including existing challenges in the sector that affect art therapists.

Museums have the potential to address a wide spectrum of health, well-being, and social needs such as healthy aging, health education, stress reduction, social isolation, pain management (linked to reduced drug consumption), enhanced mental health, increased mobility, cognitive stimulation, sociability, and employability. Although art therapy collaborations and programs have existed for decades in some museums and galleries, this work is generally unpublished. Our goal was to assemble chapters from individuals who are working to establish wellness and therapy-based programs in museums, and to illustrate that art therapy and wellness programming in these institutions is often a collaborative and interdisciplinary venture.

Different than clinical, outpatient, inpatient, school-based, and other forms of more traditional art therapy, museum art therapy happens through an interdisciplinary collaboration that might often involve education, access, and public programs. Therefore, various pedagogical, therapeutic, social practice, and accessibility approaches enrich the work of museum art therapists as they connect with concepts and knowledge from various disciplines. Art therapy does not operate as a centralized power; it, rather rhizomatically, grows by making connections with entities and power structures within the museum, as well as with outside partners.

Many art therapist roles in museums blur lines between art therapist, museum educator, and leaders in diversity, equity, inclusion, and accessibility within their institutions. No matter the roles they play, it is important to note that museum art therapists all have things in common: they are passionate about art therapy and see the potential museums have for therapeutic work.

The first part of this book provides an introduction into art therapy work in museums.

In Chapter 1, Carolyn Brown Treadon explores the history of museums, early beginnings of therapy in museums, and current applications of museum-based therapeutic work, and she offers insight into how museums can be used for therapeutic reparation. In Chapter 2, Ashley Hartman provides a deeper look at existing museum-based art therapy programming organized by population.

The second part of this book outlines several community partnership programs taking place in museums in the United States. In Chapter 3, Paige Scheinberg and Kathy Dumlao outline a partnership between the Memphis Brooks Museum of Art and an organization for juvenile offenders and discuss how the partnership has evolved over time. In Chapter 4, Mitra Reyhani Ghadim explores the collaborative nature of museum-based art therapy programming by highlighting case examples from the Queens Museum. In Chapter 5, Michelle López Torres and Mitra Reyhani Ghadim provide an example of a bi-national program for individuals with autism at the Queens Museum. In Chapter 6, Vida Sabbaghi discusses how COPE NYC partnered with the Art*Access* Program at the Queens Museum to customize internships for high school students on the autism spectrum. In Chapter 7, Sarah Pousty examines the ARTogether Program at the Children's Museum of the Arts, including the program's structure, theoretical approach, and best practices, and she looks at the program through a social justice lens. In Chapter 8, Alice Garfield highlights the development of a partnership between the Museum of Fine Arts, Boston's Artful Healing Program and Boston Children's Hospital.

The third part of the book investigates further museums' art-making spaces and studios and explores how these spaces can serve to promote healing. In Chapter 9, Rachel Shipps outlines her experience of the ways museums can be social and therapeutic spaces by examining the MakeArt Lab at the San Francisco Museum of Craft and Design. In Chapter 10, Stephen Legari discusses the Art Hive in the Montreal Museum of Fine Arts as a participatory artmaking space that empowers the public voice.

The fourth part of this book examines issues museums are grappling with in the current age of social justice: experiences of People of Color within these institutions and how to create inviting spaces that are accessible and empowering for everyone. In Chapter 11, Chloe Hayward outlines her experience with anti-oppression and anti-racist work as an art therapist, using her lived experience as a Black woman to explore art education, art therapy, and therapeutic spaces within museums. In Chapter 12, Marie Clapot presents her thoughts on how museum education concerning disability and accessibility can intersect with wellness and healing outside of an art therapy framework.

The fifth and final part of this book provides readers with practical tools and applications for utilizing museum collections in therapeutic work.

In Chapter 13, Lauren Daugherty provides an overview of how individuals make meaning from objects and discusses the process of selecting museum artworks to use in art therapy groups and individual sessions. In Chapter 14, Lauren Daugherty and Mitra Reyhani Ghadim provide examples of strategies to prompt discussion, exploration, and healing utilizing museum artworks.

1 The Power of Museums for Therapeutic Reparation

Carolyn Brown Treadon

Introduction

The use of the museum as a therapeutic resource has only recently emerged across disciplines. One of the earliest published studies (Silverman, 1989) led to increased understanding of the benefits museums could offer for diverse populations across multiple modalities. This chapter will explore a brief contextual history of museums, the early beginnings of museums being used for therapeutic processes, and foundational therapeutic uses, explore current applications with various populations, and offer insight into the use of museums for therapeutic reparation across disciplines.

Brief History

The 17th century saw the emergence of the modern concept of the museum with the opening of private collections to members of the community (Ambrose & Paine, 1993). Collections were a sign of social status; the greater the collection, the more prestige an individual attained. Museums emerged in the 18th century as institutions founded on the mission to preserve and display objects to the public (Hein, 1998). The major expansion of museums into significant public institutions occurred in the nineteenth century, where their traditional role was to preserve, document, research, and educate. It was through this education that museums sought to bring enlightenment and culture to patrons (Kaplan, Bardwell, & Slakter, 1993).

Early educational opportunities were provided to the public through special events, lectures, programming, and outreach (Hein, 1998). Items on display were labeled, including detailed descriptions when available, to enhance viewer experiences. The expansion of museum services was a response to increased awareness that the welfare of individuals was the responsibility of governmental agencies. Museums were seen as a way to provide access and education to diverse classes, leading to increased overall well-being and appreciation of the benefits of modernization. It is this foundation that led Silverman (2010) to assert that museums have always been "institutions of social service" (p. 24).

DOI: 10.4324/9781003014386-1

This mission is reflected in the mission of the American Alliance of Museums (AAM, 2020), the major accrediting agency of museums in the United States. Since its inception in 1906, the AAM has supported broad access to its institutions. As identified in the most recent strategic plan, it believes that, "museums educate and inspire, nourish minds and spirits, enrich lives and create healthy communities" (n.p.), with their strength lying in the diversity of the people represented and the breadth of museums they engage.

Similarly, the International Council of Museums (ICOM), founded in 1964, has sought the protection of cultural and natural heritage and views museums as establishments dedicated to the "service of society" (ICOM, 2020). As the world has evolved, its mission has simultaneously expanded to include the potential of museums' knowledge and resources to reach out to vulnerable groups in their communities, promote intercultural dialogue, provide experiential learning, and incorporate programs that tap into the benefits of culture.

Fundamental Functions of Museums

To accomplish their collective missions, museums must first be perceived as having more to offer than the preservation and display of objects (Treadon, Rosal, & Thompson Wylder, 2006; Treadon, 2016). In addition, museums must expand their definition of the typical museum visitor to include those from diverse backgrounds and cultures and with diverse socioeconomic status and abilities (Treadon et al., 2006; Treadon, 2016; Hein, 1998; Silverman 2010). Museums have the potential to inspire hope, promote healing, inspire lives, and lead to a better world (Silverman, 2010). This is accomplished through serving individuals by creating close partnerships with families and groups within society. These groups constitute the foundation of communities and society at large.

When individuals enter the museum space, a relationship unfolds between the visitor(s) and their experiences (Jensen, 1982). This experience is shaped though the interplay between what the individual brings with them – their lived experiences – and the museum. For meaningful interaction to occur, the museum environment must actively engage the individual and reward their attention. There must be a connection to something familiar, a place, event, emotion, or experience (Hein, 1998). This is a space where personal meaning-making can occur (Silverman, 2010).

Through strategic use of exhibitions, museums can serve many functions, including, but not limited to, the exhibition of historical artifacts, increasing community education and awareness, and therapeutic programming (Peacock, 2012). To accomplish this, museums must determine current functioning and identify what changes may lead to more engagement opportunities. Silverman et al. (2012) undertook a study to identify hinderances that existed in the successful engagement and inclusivity for patrons of interactive museums. They identified three areas that had a direct impact: modifications to the environment, innovative programming, and personnel training. Addressing these areas can lead to increased community engagement, opening the museum up as an inclusive space for diverse audiences (Hein, 1998; Rochford, 2017).

Mangione (2018) saw the role of the museum as a co-facilitator within the treatment framework as an evolution rather than an innovation of practice. For centuries, individuals have sought museums, including outdoor spaces such as gardens, for solace and rejuvenation. These institutions were seen as a way to escape, for a period of time, the stressors of daily life. Sustained mental effort leads to what Kaplan et al. (1993) discussed as directed attention fatigue (DAF). DAF leads to increased distractibility, impatience, irritability, and unnecessary risk taking due to impaired reasoning. To compensate, individuals must have access to a restorative environment.

Restorative environments must possess four criteria (Kaplan et al., 1993). First, *being away*, a physical relocation from normal environments. Second is *extent* – being in a physical space that is extended in time and space, providing an opportunity for a state of flow. *Fascination* is the third component; one's attention must be engaged in a meaningful way. Last is *compatibility* – the encounter must align with one's purposes. The more properties met, the greater the chance for restoration. Museums can address all four of these criteria. The story behind artifacts or art imagery and engaging exhibitions can facilitate the personal connections, leading to greater engagement and restoration (Ioannides, 2017).

In her foundational research, Silverman (1989) explored the therapeutic use of the museum with a family, leading to her continued research into the museum as an agent of social work (Silverman, 2010). She identified eight distinct therapeutic purposes museums offer:

1. Interactive experiences and social relationships
2. Communication as meaning-making
3. The meaning of things
4. Human needs
5. Outcomes and changing
6. Relationship benefits and social capital
7. Social change
8. Culture change (Silverman, 2010, p. 14).

Salom (2011, 2015) identified additional benefits to include artistic diversity, architectural boundaries, the collective nature of the artifacts and art imagery, interpersonal exchanges, and changes in scenery. Additionally, he identified four roles museums can fill in treatment: the museum as co-leader (keeping the focus on goal attainment in the environment), the museum as group (the knowledge of the group of artifacts/art imagery), the museum as self (representing wholeness in an organized manner), and the museum as environment (interrelation between time, space, and objects).

During a museum visit, interactions happen at varying degrees with family members, museum staff, other patrons, and society at large (Silverman, 2010). Museum learning and engagement are social processes – they do not happen in isolation (Hein, 1998). They challenge individuals to expand their views and lead to increases in self-esteem, confidence, and creativity through increased intellectual stimulation and breaking away from normal routine (Hein, 1998; Ioannides, 2017). These benefits, which promote well-being, are a direct result of decreased social isolation. Mental and psychological wellness can be restored in the peace and calmness of the museum (Kaplan et al., 1993). Museums serve to help with identity formation, development of friendships, and facilitation of social bonds between individuals, families, and cultures (Silverman, 2010).

Across disciplines, the knowledge of the therapeutic benefits of museums has expanded and been embraced (Mangione, 2018). Museums provide a sense of normalcy as a nonclinical setting for wellness (Coles & Harrison, 2018; Thomson et al. 2011, 2018). As a community-based resource, the focus is on promoting overall psychological well-being (Ioannides, 2017). To fulfill this, museums must be able to attract and retain attention through relating to the lived experiences individuals bring with them (Jensen, 1982). Art imagery and artifacts reflect collective human experiences allowing individuals to relate to what they are viewing, reducing feelings of isolation and detachment. The addition of small group discussions further promotes social engagement, reducing social isolation (D'Cunha et al., 2019). For both observers and creators, engaging in responsive activities can lead to increased mood and other psychological states, impacting overall physical health (Newpoff, Melnyk, & Neale, 2018).

Museums offer many inherent benefits as therapeutic settings. They challenge individuals' perceptions about art, history, and culture (Rochford, 2017). Through processing these challenging concepts within the museum setting, increased insight and self-awareness are fostered. To best provide the scaffolding needed for these experiences, there must be an understanding about meanings visitors create using their museum experiences – those that are ordinary and those that are extraordinary (Hein, 1998). Through enhanced communication with museum professionals, other professionals, and individuals, museums' roles as agents of social change continue to evolve (Silverman et al., 2012; Silverman 2010).

Early Uses of the Museum for Therapeutic Reparation

The Queens Museum in New York developed the Please Touch Initiative for individuals who were blind or low vision to engage in art education in the early 1980s (Reyhani Dejkameh & Shipps, 2019). This provided the foundation for Art*Access* to expand its reach to include programming to support those living with mental illness. As programming expanded, Art*Access* began including internships for art education and art therapy students, who learned the importance of adapting to the needs of participants to provide meaningful engagement in the museum environment. Programming expanded to include nursing homes, children's hospitals, schools, and psychiatric centers. Vocational training for individuals with disabilities was developed in response to societal need. The focus remained on social acceptance in the least restrictive environment.

Silverman (1989) and Williams (1994) were two of the earlier researchers to publish about the potential of museums. Silverman (1989) sought to explore the potential relationship between the museum and family therapy. Engaging the family in a museum visit helps facilitate social interaction and communication through decision-making. Conflicts must be navigated. Silverman presented a theoretical framework for future research on the use of museums as therapeutic tools.

Williams (1994) investigated the role of the museum for personal exploration. As a museum educator, he sought alternative ways an art museum could engage visitors who were hesitant to discuss the connection between art objects and life experiences. He created an experimental program employing a "personal highlights tour," where participants chose a prompt (Figure 1.1) and found a piece of art within the museum that they felt addressed the prompt, and each led a discussion on the art selected.

These are Williams's Personal Highlights Tour prompts:

1. Find a work of art that you find moving. What is it about the work that touched you?
2. Find a work of art that you find moving. What does that work have to tell you about your own life?
3. Find a work of art that seems to be calling you. Ask the work, "What do you have to tell me about my life?" Wait for a response.
4. Find a work of art that reminds you of something in your past. Think about the connection.
5. Choose a gallery and find a work of art that is most like you. What similarities do you find?
6. Find a work of art that speaks to you on an emotional level. Take time to experience it fully. . . . Be aware of changing physical sensations, fleeting thoughts, or memories.
7. Find a work of art that speaks to you on an emotional level. Take time to experience it fully. How would you describe your feelings?
8. Choose a gallery and find a work that you think is most likely to evoke a similar emotional response in everyone who comes to see it. Think about the reasons for your choice.
9. Find a work that gives you clues about the artist's personality, values, or feelings. How are they communicated through the work of art?

Other early programming explored the use of museums for marginalized populations. Arts for Health at the National Gallery of Australia sought to provide benefits for individuals with chronic illnesses (Winn, nd). Similarly, the Contemporary Museum in Honolulu provided tours and responsive art-making workshops for individuals suffering from traumatic brain injuries (Lobos, nd). The McMichael Canadian Art Collection Gallery developed therapeutic programs housed in the gallery that combined art therapy and museum education for self-actualization and social involvement (Hartman & Brown, 2016), including programs for individuals living with HIV/AIDS and troubled youth.

Museums visits have led to increased self-esteem, self-acceptance, self-growth, social awareness, decreased symptomology, and creativity. Stiles and Mermer-Welly (1998) explored the role of poor self-esteem in early teen pregnancy, and Alter-Muri, S. (1996) explored the use of art history and art reproductions that served as a catalyst for clients seeking out museums to enhance their treatment. Linesch (2004) collaborated with the director of special exhibits at the Museum of Tolerance in Los Angeles to facilitate workshops in response to a special exhibition of the work of Friedl Dicker-Brandeis, an artist who taught art to hundreds of children in the Terezin concentration camp and ultimately perished in Auschwitz. The workshops provided opportunities for patrons to engage with and respond to the exhibit.

Based on the work of these earlier researchers, a pilot project was developed between the Florida State University Museum of Fine Art and the graduate art therapy program to assess how the museum could function as a therapeutic tool (Treadon et al., 2006; Treadon, 2016). Partnering with a local school that served children with severe emotional and behavioral disorders, family was identified as the theme owing to the evolution of the definition of families in modern society. Students engaged in sessions that included works of art from the museum's collection at the school prior to attending the museum and engaging in a modified "personal highlights tour." All encounters included responsive art. At the conclusion of the pilot program, students selected a completed work of art they wanted to include in a gallery exhibition at the museum.

One participant, who had been quiet but engaged in the process, chose his self-portrait. It was completed in response to William Walmsley's *Self Portrait* (2001). In discussing the image with the group, he noted the figure did not have a mouth (Figure 1.1). He requested a pencil and drew a mouth, indicating the image was now complete (Figure 1.2). One may infer from this that participating in the museum experience allowed him to feel he had more of a voice (Treadon et al., 2006; Treadon, 2016).

These experiences have laid the foundation for the many current programs that exist in museums and galleries throughout the world. They have taught us that the success of museum visits can be assessed on the connection individuals make between old and new ideas in response to the artifacts and art imagery they encounter. Collaborations must exist between museum educators and staff and those providing psychological or physiological support (Treadon et al., 2006; Livingston, Fiterman Persin, & Del Signore, 2016; Silverman, 2010).

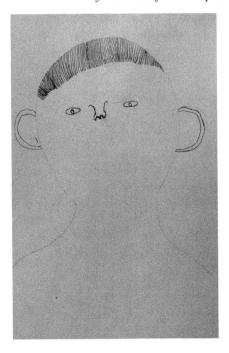

Figure 1.1 Original self-portrait without mouth

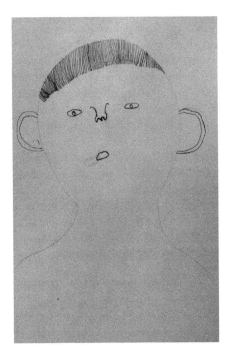

Figure 1.2 Revised self-portrait with mouth

Together, these collaborative partnerships help to create safe spaces needed for individuals to make connections between what they are experiencing and their own lives.

Current Applications of Museums for Therapeutic Reparation

There has been an increase in the use of museums as 'social prescriptions.' These prescriptions include interpersonal engagement, physical activity, personal exploration, and creative encounters and are in response to delinquency, physical ailments, and psychological needs. This rise has re-ignited the use of museums as community-based assets that have social value (Thomson et al., 2018). Over the last decade, the role of museums as agents of well-being has led to alignments with healthcare professionals for addressing Alzheimer's/dementia, traumatic brain injury, post-traumatic stress, and more (Rosenblatt, 2014).

Alzheimer's and Dementia

There are many benefits of engaging with museum objects for people living with dementia (PLWD). By viewing, experiencing, and discussing art, individuals experienced a decrease in depressive symptoms, an increase in self-reported quality of life, and increased cognitive functions, including verbal fluency (D'Cunha et al., 2019). Following visits to the National Gallery of Australia, participants were observed to be happier, with increased laughter and engagement between sessions. Similar outcomes were found by the Art in the Moment program serving PLWD and their caregivers (Livingston et al., 2016). Participants reported decreased feelings of isolation, increased mood for the PLWD and their caregiver, increased personal validation through socialization, and a reported benefit of engagement in activities that were nonclinical.

An open-air museum in the United Kingdom took a different approach, creating an 8-week group for men LWD (Kindleysides & Biglands, 2015). The group did not focus on the cognitive impairments, but rather on the participants' strengths to encourage active and full participation. Tasks were intentionally developed to take several weeks and require different ability levels. Traditional tools from the museum were used. Participants reported benefits in increased engagement and socialization and feeling a sense of belonging and purpose.

The Creative Aging program at the Phillips Collection provided encounters for older adults and care providers to participate in group discussions on museum artifacts and create responsive pieces (Rosenblatt, 2014). Through this process, interpersonal connections were fostered, connections between participants and objects were formed, and participants developed an increases sense of purpose and accomplishment. Thomson et al. (2018) found similar outcomes in participants who were identified as at risk based on social isolation. The 10-week programs occurred at various museums across London and Kent. Upon conclusion, participants discussed enjoyment from engaging with curators and other staff, handling objects, and learning new skills and knowledge. Some participants, however, expressed frustration with exhaustion when navigating the museum spaces and fatigue with the creative process.

For some older individuals, change can be challenging. Salom (2011) worked with a local care facility for older adults in Colombia (<70) to participate in a museum-based visit to help them become open to new experiences. Visiting the Museo Arqueologico Casa del Marqués de San Jorge provided a change in location and routine and an opportunity to engage with and reflect upon historical artifacts and promoted increased social connection. Following the visit, participants engaged in artmaking, and most found the process beneficial, requesting to keep their productions.

Hospitals

When in hospital, patients are often faced with many challenges including a loss of autonomy. Thomson et al. (2011) found that handling museum object reproductions had an effect on inpatients at University College Hospital in London. Participants were provided a choice of objects and were able to interact with the chosen object, followed by a discussion. Participants reported an increase in positive emotions, feelings of well-being and happiness, and a reduction in negative mood. These changes led to an increase in positive relationships with other patients and staff.

Similar results were found in the Le Louvre à L'Hôpital program, which brought the museum to the hospital (Monsuez et al., 2019). Reproductions of famous artworks were taken to the hospital and displayed in public areas, including dining areas, gardens, and public spaces. Patients in chosen areas (rehabilitation, treatment for addiction, long-term geriatric and palliative care) were also able to select art to be displayed in their rooms as their expected stay was longer. Additionally, patients on these units also tended to have increased levels of anxiety and depression.

While in the hospital, participants were encouraged to engage in guided tours that included interactive discussions encouraging personal connections. Participants reported a reduction in anxiety and overall satisfaction with the program. However, patients who were able to visit the Louvre on a day trip reported a decrease in satisfaction due to fatigue and an increase in anxiety from being overwhelmed. Because of the benefits in the hospital, staff were trained to continue the program in the absence of museum staff (Monsuez et al., 2019).

Mental Health

The Montreal Museum of Fine Art partnered with the Douglas University Institute's Eating Disorder Program to provide adjunctive treatment for participants (Thaler et al., 2017). Weekly trips to the museum were optional, in addition to other standardized care. Participants engaged in a guided tour of selected works with museum staff and created reflective art that culminated in a group discussion with an art therapist. Benefits reported included that the program was a pleasing activity that allowed participants to enter a new setting, offering distraction from their typical thoughts. Reflective artmaking allowed for increased creativity and self-expression. Many appreciated the choices they were able to make in the process. Museum staff engaged with participants, helping them acquire new knowledge and perspectives.

Salom (2011) found that adults with mental illness benefited from the museum encounter. Following a self-guided tour of the Museo Arqueologico Casa del Marqués de San Jorge in Bogotá, Colombia, which included sketching items of interest, participants were provided space to create. They were asked to reflect on their sketches and items they found interesting and to create a clay sculpture. Through processing their sculptures, participants demonstrated an ability to connect artifacts to their personal lives, leading to increased self-awareness and understanding.

Coles and Harrison (2018) provided arts psychotherapy to young adults (18–25) with persistent mental illness in programs at the Gloucester Life Museum and the Museum of Gloucester. The museums were chosen for this demographic owing to the nonclinical setting and their ability to foster independence in participants by helping them connect with something outside of the mental health spectrum. The 18-week program was split between the two museums, with each visit lasting 90 minutes. Each encounter followed the same format, with check-in, museum exploration, creative response, and discussion. Following the conclusion of the program, participants reported increased self-understanding, increased formation of relationships, encouragement for ongoing social inclusion, and increased creativity.

Displaced and Migrant Populations

Displaced and migrant populations face many challenges when relocating. In helping them adjust to the new environment without losing their identity, museums can function as a welcoming agent (Salom, 2015). Contextually, museums can offer a connection to the 'motherland' and help individuals draw on the arts, as a familiar form of expression, to help facilitate adjustment. Internally displaced indigenous women participated in a program at the Museo del Oro in Bogotá, Colombia. With the goal of emotional expression, the experience led the participants to express and honor their own cultural identity in a safe, nonjudgmental way.

Veterans

In their mission to respond to community needs, museums have the potential to address difficult topics. Veterans face many challenges when deployed, upon return, and when dealing with traumas experienced. The inability to connect with others who have faced similar events can exacerbate challenges. An artist, with guidance from veterans, sought to create an installation to help increase visitors' awareness of the traumas experienced in war (Ruehrwein, 2013). *Out of Here*, housed in the Institute of Contemporary Art in Boston, recreated a mortar attack in Iraq. Throughout the 5-month installation, feedback collected indicated that the project led to increased dialogue and understanding for the public and enabled a venue to address an important community issue.

Debilitating stress can hinder veterans from reintegrating into civilian life. Finding appropriate community resources to support their needs can be challenging; balancing the potential for good with limits is even more challenging. The Chicago Botanic Garden sought to find this balance in working with the Veterans Project (Kreski, 2016). Through staff development training and collaboration with therapeutic support staff, a half-day retreat was developed for veterans and their therapists that included structured and unstructured activities. Veterans reported that the environment felt safe and welcoming, a place where they did not feel different, and they were able to escape while there, leading to reduced stress, anxiety, and hypervigilance. Use of a botanical garden as a therapeutic space reinforces their historical purpose of providing health and wellness (Mangione, 2018).

Future Directions

Museums have been taking on an ever-evolving role as agents of social change and wellness. They possess the potential to provide "universal social service" (Silverman, 2010, p. 142). Through embracing social inclusion, museums have the potential to enhance the development of social cohesion (Ioannides, 2017; Kreski, 2016). They provide an environment that is supportive in which to address and confront difficult topics and they impact overall well-being through providing opportunities for engagement with artifacts in an interactive environment (Ioannides, 2017; Kindleysides & Biglands, 2015; Salom, 2011; Silverman, 2010).

Participation in community life is essential to overall health and wellness (Silverman et al., 2012). Throughout the process of individuals engaging with artifacts, art images, and each other, museums serve as a holding space and facilitator for personal growth, relationship building, healing, and social change (Silverman, 2010). Their resources offer untapped benefits to individuals and communities (Salom, 2011). The contents of museums may serve as conduits for self-awareness and increased insights (Thomson et al., 2018). The museums' support acts as an agent in increasing public health and wellness.

This potential must be exploited strategically. There is much to gain from partnerships, but they must be mutual and collaborative. Peacock (2012) found that, when therapeutic benefit is envisioned to further the mission and goals of a museum, innovative partnerships are more likely to be successful. Through identifying community needs, partnerships can develop (Kreski, 2016). Additionally, bringing the museum into alternative spaces requires collaboration and flexibility. The benefits of arts-related practices in healthcare settings have increased overall well-being and decreased anxiety and stress (Thomson et al., 2011). All participants must clearly communicate goals, needs, aspirations, and limitations while also being willing to listen to and learn from each other (Treadon et al., 2006; Treadon, 2016; Rochford, 2017; Ruehrwein, 2013; Salom, 2011, 2015; Silverman, 2010).

For therapeutic benefit to occur, safety must be established. It is the role of the facilitator to create a climate that promotes full engagement in the process and containment for difficult emotions (Williams, 1994). Feeling comfortable and able to navigate space can significantly impact the restorative value of the museum (Kaplan et al., 1993; Kindleysides & Biglands, 2015; Salom, 2011). Providing choices, when they are appropriate, can increase a feeling of control for participants in an unfamiliar environment (Jensen, 1982). Retaining the nonclinical environment is crucial. Artifacts, art images, and other elements must be strategically chosen to best meet the needs of participants (Salom, 2011). The frequency, duration, location within the museum, and timing of visits are essential. For some, the busy and, at times, loud museum environment can be overwhelming and nontherapeutic. There are many variables that must be considered to help facilitate a successful encounter.

Globally, doctors and researchers are prescribing museum visits, finding that an increase in overall wellness leads to an increase in physical and mental health (Hunt, 2019; Solly, 2019). For patients with chronic pain, a prescription to the museum is providing relief and increased quality of life (Remiorz, 2018). Those living with dementia are increasingly being referred to museums for treatment, finding that the visits improve overall quality of life (Elbaor, 2019). In New York, minor offenders can participate in an art class to avoid jail time (Bishara, 2019). Early results indicate a decrease in recidivism for repeat offences. "Art*Access* has grown into a nationally replicated model designed to allow audiences of all abilities to enjoy a personal connection to art and cultural institutions" (Queens Museum, n.d.). These programs demonstrate the versatility of museums in serving the greater good of communities.

Conclusion

Museums have a long-standing history as social service agents. Though initially seen as institutions to preserve, document, research, and educate, museums have emerged as powerful allies in reparation and wellness across the globe. By creating partnerships with different organizations, museums have expanded their missions to be ever more inclusive of diverse patrons, broadening the definition of who museums are established to serve. Through understanding the needs of diverse individuals, strong communication with museum curators, educators, and other museum professionals, and connecting goals to museum resources, art therapists can create opportunities to positively impact individuals' overall mental, physical, and spiritual health for enhanced treatment.

References

Alter-Muri, S. (1996). Dali to Beuys: Incorporating art history in art therapy treatment plans. *Art Therapy: Journal of the American Art Therapy Association, 13*(2), 102–107. https://doi.org/10.1080/07421656.1996.10759203

Ambrose, T. & Pain, C. (1993). *Museum basics*. Routledge.

American Alliance of Museums. (2020). *Strategic Plan.* Retrieved from: www.aam-us. org/programs/about-aam/american-alliance-of-museums-strategic-plan/

Bishara, H. (2019, October 24). Minor offenders can substitute jail time with an art class at the Brooklyn Museum. *Hyperallergic*. Retrieved from: https://hyperallergic. com/522716/minor-offenders-can-substitute-jail-time-for-an-art-class-at-the-brooklyn-museum/?fbclid=IwAR0EEr1OG1gH8ZfDaAmPY9mcRQ5fIWz15UbDkdYPMUc IiEFJGXMJN7ioFOI

Coles, A. & Harrison, F. (2018). Tapping into museums for art psychotherapy: An evaluation of a pilot group for young adults. *International Journal of Art Therapy, 23*(3), 115–124. https://doi.org/10.1080/17454832.2017.1380056

D'Cunha, N. M., Mckune, A. J., Isbel, S., Kellett, J., Georgousopoulou, E. N. & Naumovski, N. (2019). Psychophysiological responses in people living with dementia after an art gallery intervention: An exploratory study. *Journal of Alzheimer's Disease, 72*(2), 549–562. https://doi.org/10.3233/JAD-190784

Elbaor, C. (2019, November 28). Researchers have found that visiting art museums can offer significant relief for people living with dementia. *ArtNet News*. Retrieved from: https://news.artnet.com/art-world/research-dementia-art-museums-1718127?fbclid= IwAR359tHDj9LrH9iHjEr41gw6T-4RanMmNMoys6vzIX8ThwFq420hkI0we80

Hartman, A. & Brown, S. (2016). Synergism through therapeutic visual arts. In V. C. Bryan & J. L. Bird (Eds.), *Healthcare community synergism between patients, practitioners, and researchers (advances in medical diagnosis, treatment, and care)* (29–48). IGI Global.

Hein, G. E. (1998). *Learning in the museum*. Routledge.

Hunt, K. (2019, December 18). Visit museums or art galleries and you may live longer, new research suggests. *CNNstyle*. Retrieved from: www.cnn.com/style/article/art-longevity-wellness/index.html?fbclid=IwAR3G9rIMfEbdfhk5wzC51Cu4ZW4yyw a3uDXai2UxnjxUeRizoG7srbPheH8

International Council of Museums. (2020). *Missions and objectives*. Retrieved from: https://icom.museum/en/about-us/missions-and-objectives/

Ioannides, E. (2017). Museums as therapeutic environments in the contribution of art therapy. *Museum International, 68*(271–272), 98–109.

Jensen, N. E. (1982). Children, teenagers, and adults in museums: A developmental perspective. *Museum News, 60*, 25–30.

Kaplan, S., Bardwell, L. V. & Slakter, D. B. (1993). The museum as a restorative environment. *Environment and Behavior, 25*(6), 725–742.

Kindleysides, M. & Biglands, E. (2015). "Thinking outside the box, and making it too": Piloting an occupational therapy group at an open air museum. *Arts and Health, 7*(3), 271–278. https://doi.org/10.1080/17533015.2015.1061569

Kreski, B. (2016). Healing and empowering veterans in a botanic garden. *Journal of Museum Education, 41*(2), 110–115. https://doi.org/10.1080/10598650.2016.1169734

Linesch, D. (2004). Art therapy at the Museum of Tolerance: Responses to the life and work of Friedl Dicker-Brandeis. *The Arts in Psychotherapy, 31*(2), 57–66. https://doi.org/10.1016/j.aip.2004.02.004

Livingston, L., Fiterman Persin, G., & Del Signore, D. (2016). Art in the moment: Evaluating a therapeutic wellness program for people with dementia and their care partners. *Journal of Museum Education, 41*(2), 100–109. https://doi.org/10.1080/10598650.2016.1169735

Lobos, I. (nd). *Fine art: Good therapy*. The Contemporary Museum in Honolulu.

Mangione, G. (2018). The art and nature of health: A study of therapeutic practice in museums. *Sociology of Health & Illness, 40*(2), 283–296. https://doi.org/10.1111/1467-9566.12618

Monsuez, J., François, V., Ratiney, R., Trinchet, I., Polomeni, P., Sebbane, G., Muller, S., Litout, M., Castagno, C. & Frandji, D. (2019). Museum moving to inpatients: Le Louvre à L'Hôpital. *International Journal of Environmental Research and Public Health, 16*(2), 206–212. https://doi.org/10.3390/ijerph16020206

Newpoff, L. D., Melnyk, B. M., & Neale, S. (2018). Creative wellness: A missing link in boosting well-being. *American Nurse Today, 13*(8), 11–13.

Peacock, K. (2012). Museum education and art therapy: Exploring an innovative partnership. *Art Therapy, 29*(3), 133–137. https://doi.org/10.1080/07421656.2012.701604

Queens Museum. (n.d.). Art*Access*. Retrieved from: https://queensmuseum.org/art-access

Remiorz, R. (2018, October 12). Doctors to prescribe museum visits to help patients "escape from their own pain." *CBC News*. www.cbc.ca/news/canada/montreal/montreal-museum-fine-arts-medecins-francophone-art-museum-therapy-1.4859936

Reyhani Dejkameh, M. & Shipps, R. (2019) From please touch to Art*Access*: The expansion of a museum-based art therapy program. *Art Therapy*, 35(4), 211–217. https://doi.org/10.1080/07421656.2018.1540821

Rochford, J. (2017). Art therapy and art museum education: A visitor focused collaboration. *Art Therapy, 34*(4), 209–214. https://doi.org/10.1080/07421656.2017.1383787

Rosenblatt, B. (2014). Museum education and art therapy: Promoting wellness in older adults. *Journal of Museum Education, 39*(3), 293–301.

Ruehrwein, B. J. (2013). The art museum as trauma clinic: A veteran's story. *Museum and Social Issues, 8*(1&2), 36–46. https://doi.org/10.1179/1559689313Z.0000000005

Salom, A. (2011). Reinventing the setting: Art therapy in museums. *The Arts in Psychotherapy, 38*(2), 81–85. https://doi.org/10.1016/j.aip.2010.12.004

Salom, A. (2015). Weaving potential space and acculturation: Art therapy at the museum. *Journal of Applies Arts & Health, 6*(2), 47–62. https://doi.org/10.1386/jaah.6.1.47_1

Silverman, F., Bartley, B., Cohn, E., Kanics, I. M. & Walsh, L. (2012). Occupational therapy partnerships with museums: Creating inclusive environments that promote participation and belonging. *The International Journal of the Inclusive Museum, 4*(4), 15–30. http://dx.doi.org/10.18848/1835-2014/CGP/v04i04/44384

Silverman, L. (1989). "Johnny showed us the butterflies": The museum as a family therapy tool. *Marriage and Family Review, 13*(3–4), 131–150. https://doi.org/10.1300/J002v13n03_08

Silverman, L. (2010). *The social work of museums*. Routledge

Solly, M. (2019, October 22). Canadian doctors will soon be able to prescribe museum visits as treatment. *Smithsonian Magazine*. Retrieved from: www.smithsonianmag.com/smart-news/canadian-doctors-will-soon-be-able-prescribe-museum-visits-180970599/

Stiles, G. J. & Mermer-Welly, M. J. (1998). Children having children: Art therapy in a community-based early adolescent pregnancy program. *Art Therapy*, *15*(3), 165–176. doi:10.1080/07421656.1989.10759319

Thaler, L., Drapeau, C., Leclerc, J., Lajeunesse, M., Cottier, D., Kahan, E., Ferenczy, N. & Steiger, H. (2017). An adjunctive, museum-based art therapy experience in the treatment of women with severe eating disorders. *The Arts in Psychotherapy*, *56*, 1–6. https://doi.org/10.1016/j.aip.2017.08.002

Thomson, L. J., Ander, E., Menon, U., Lanceley, A. & Chatterjee, H. (2011). Evaluating the therapeutic effects of museum object handling with hospital patients: A review and initial trial of well-being measures. *Journal of Applied Arts and Health*, *2*(1), 37–56. https://doi.org/10.1386/jaah.2.1.37_1

Thomson, L. J., Lockyer, B., Camic, P. M., & Chatterjee, H. J. (2018). Effects of a museum-based social prescription intervention on quantitative measures of psychological wellbeing in older adults. *Perspectives in Public Health*, *138*(1), 28–38. https://doi.org/10.1177/1757913917737563

Treadon, C. B. (2016). Bringing art therapy into museums. In D. Gussak & M. Rosal (Eds.), *The Wiley handbook of art therapy* (487–496). John Wiley.

Treadon, C. B., Rosal, M. & Thompson Wylder, V. D. (2006). Opening the doors of art museums for therapeutic process. *The Arts in Psychotherapy*, *33*(4), 288–301. https://doi.org/10.1016/j.aip.2006.03.003

Williams, R. (1994). *Honoring the museum visitors' personal associations and emotional responses to art: Work towards a model for educators*. Paper presented to the faculty at Harvard University.

Winn, P. (nd). *Arts for health: Art therapy at the National Gallery of Australia*.

2 Exploring Museum-based Art Therapy

A Summary of Existing Programs

Ashley Hartman

Introduction

Museum-based art therapy (MBAT) is a community-based practice that has evolved and expanded through the work of several art therapists since the 1990s. Bringing art therapy into the museum presents the potential to improve quality of life for diverse client populations (Linesch, 2004; Salom, 2011; Treadon, Rosal, & Thompson Wylder, 2006). Several programs have used the museum and gallery space for different therapeutic objectives, and they have been structured and facilitated in different ways based on the theoretical approach of the art therapist, the mission and needs of museum programming, and the therapeutic benefits being addressed. This chapter will outline the nature of existing MBAT programs that have been published in art therapy literature. The programs outlined in the subsequent tables have been organized based on population type and emphasis of the therapeutic implications of using the museum as a space for creative art interventions. MBAT practice spans a broad range of client populations within various community organizations. The programs outlined in the table were highlighted in an art therapy-related publication with a clear description of the MBAT session and protocol. Art therapists, individually or collaboratively, facilitated the sessions in each program.

In 2012, Peacock outlined several partnerships that had taken place between art therapy and museum education collaborations. Some of these programs included less detailed descriptions of the programming and/or lack of publications and scholarly literature documenting these works. Since then, art therapists have increasingly written about their work. In 2016, art therapy authors began to explore the theoretical and practical potential of utilizing the museum as a space for art therapy (Treadon, 2016; Hamil, 2016; Ioannides, 2016). The progress and contributions from such art therapists have led to a summation of the information presented in the tables below, which highlight the types and scopes of programs with rich description of the art therapy protocols and therapeutic implications central to the work for each client group or issue.

The first four tables presented outline MBAT programs that have been designed for developmental age groups. The second set of tables outlines

DOI: 10.4324/9781003014386-2

Table 2.1 MBAT Programs Designed for Diverse Adolescent Populations

Authors Museum, Program Title & Collaborating Partnerships	Population(s) Served	MBAT Program Structure and Protocol	Therapeutic Intentions
Hartman, 2019 Florida State University Museum of Fine Arts (MoFA) and Art Therapy Doctoral Dissertation Project	Adolescents ages 13–17 Diagnosis of high-functioning autism (HFA) 3 female, 1 male	Narrative art therapy groups held over 16 weeks; 2 hours each session held twice weekly. 1. Meet and greet 2. 20-minute free choice gallery exploration or guided object visit 3. 20-minute therapeutic discussion 4. 60–70-minute artmaking experience and processing. Connect to themes from: *The Art of the Educator*, the Watercolor Society, the *Blacklight Exhibition*, and the MFA Graduating Artist exhibition My Own Expression, a co-curated client exhibition, was hosted in the museum; family/community members were invited	Explore adolescent identity development, socioemotional development Enhance communication and self-expression Promote sensory integration, problem-solving and decision-making, developing a narrative that depicts understanding of self and diagnosis

(Continued)

Table 2.1 (Continued)

Authors Museum, Program Title & Collaborating Partnerships	Population(s) Served	MBAT Program Structure and Protocol	Therapeutic Intentions
Marxen, 2009 MACBA Contemporary Art Museum of Barcelona and Miquel Tarradell Secondary School	Adolescents ages 13–16 Challenges with social skills and demonstrated behavioral problems in school	Feminist, critical theory, gender technology, urban history, political immigration, and economy framework 1. Art psychotherapist used the artists Sophie Calle, Krzysztof Wodiczko, and clinical work of Lygia Clark to connect to personal lives of clients 2. Explored themes related to social justice, environmentalism, and sociopolitical issues 3. Art therapy workshops focused on creative process	Provide an outlet for self-expression Provide a safe space to explore relational issues Promote social skills and prosocial behavior
Treadon et al., 2006 Florida State University Museum of Fine Arts (MoFA) and Graduate Art Therapy Program	Adolescents ages 12–14 Severe emotional and behavioral disorders, depression, obsessive-compulsive tendencies, and hyperactivity 6 male, 1 female	Art therapy sessions focused on family theme. Seven sessions held off-site with two visits to the museum 1. Carefully selected objects based on family theme. Museum objects (self-portraits) brought off-site for a viewing 2. Artmaking sessions reflected on personal experiences, thoughts, and emotions about the family system Co-curated client exhibition: The Family Experience	Expand services to diverse client populations in the community Enhance prosocial behavior, engagement, self-confidence, motivation, and autonomy Decrease resistance and problematic behavior

Linesch, 2004 Museum of Tolerance in Los Angeles, California, & Loyola Marymount University Art Therapy Program	Middle school participants and family members	1. Museum tours of Anne Frank documents, Friedl-Dicker-Brandeis and Children of Terezin, and Finding our Families: Finding Ourselves 2. Explored themes related to privacy or feeling boxed in, like Anne Frank 3. 2-hour art therapy workshops at the museum connected to the themes of the museum exhibit. Art therapy themes coincided with exhibitions. Created papier mâché masks and small boxes with collage words	Provide an outlet for self-expression. Facilitate resiliency through creative process Learn from the stories of inspirational historical figures Help define personal identities, explore self in context of immediate families
Stiles and Mermer-Welly, 1998 The Toledo Museum of Art and Toledo Public Schools Early Adolescent Pregnancy Program	Pregnant female adolescents with mild to moderate intellectual disabilities Ages 13–15 years old Diverse sociocultural backgrounds: 68% African American, 75% living in single-parent, female-headed household	Group art therapy, family therapy, and 90-minute weekly group art therapy sessions conducted in alternative school setting 1. Socialization and museum gallery visits using a community-based approach to talk about cultural standards of beauty 2. Artworks in the gallery were explored for specific themes associated with pregnancy. Socialization and warm-up exercise 3. Artmaking and group processing	Explore stereotypes about beauty, self-esteem, attractiveness, and family dynamics and relationships Promote self-expression, self-exploration, risk-taking Reflect on emotions, current activities, sexual attitudes/feelings, and somatic complaint of the adolescents' lives and families because of their pregnancy

programs that were designed to address a particular client issue, need, or concern. A description of the program structure, art therapy protocol, and implication of therapeutic benefits were made available for these programs.

Summary of MBAT Programs Designed for Diverse Adolescent Populations

Table 2.1 depicts MBAT programs that were designed specifically for adolescents. Each of these adolescent programs aimed to provide an outlet and space for a particular underrepresented population, including individuals with high-functioning autism (Hartman, 2019), emotional behavioral disorders (Treadon et al., 2006), aggressive behavioral issues (Marxen, 2009), pregnant teens facing self-esteem issues (Stiles & Mermer-Welly, 1998), or middle school students and family members (Linesch, 2004).

Four programs were hosted in museums in the United States, and one was hosted in Barcelona. Three museums collaborated with graduate art therapy programs, and two collaborated with community partner organizations. The structure of each program differed. Some sessions were facilitated in the museum exclusively, and others took place off-site, incorporating museum visits and/or object visit sessions into the traditional session structure.

Art therapy approaches utilized in these programs included psychotherapy, narrative approaches, family art therapy, group art therapy, and studio art therapy. Theme-based protocols were frequently used to connect the museum objects or content in exhibitions with the lives and experiences of the audience. Furthermore, therapeutic discussions aligned with the needs of each population being served.

The family theme was emphasized throughout several of the programs mentioned (Hartman, 2019; Linesch, 2004; Treadon et al., 2006; Stiles & Mermer-Welly, 1998). Many of the art therapy experientials addressed issues such as exploration of the self in the context of the family system, as well as perception of family relationships and dynamics. In the case of Marxen's (2009) group, a focus on social justice themes offered an outlet for adolescents to express personal responses to controversial issues, both through art viewing in the gallery and artmaking sessions with the art psychotherapist. One program mentioned applying an object-focused approach that explored museum objects to enhance self-confidence and to understand emotions and feelings about the object.

Summary of MBAT Programs Designed for Young Adult Populations

Since 1996, Alter-Muri has incorporated trips to the museum galleries as part of therapeutic treatment plans. In the museum, young adult programming has been developed to enhance the quality of lives of young adult population individuals with autism (Legari, personal communication, 2019; Reyhani Dejkameh &

Table 2.2 MBAT Programs Designed for Diverse Young Adult Populations

Authors Museum, Program Title & Collaborating Partnerships	Population(s) Served	MBAT Program Structure and Protocol	Therapeutic Intentions
Coles, Harrison, & Todd, 2019 Museum of Gloucester and Gloucester Life Museum	Young adults 18–25 with complex mental health difficulties Groups included 6–10 participants	Art psychotherapy groups over 20 weeks used exhibitions/objects from prehistory, natural history, and decorative arts, and contemporary art 1. Check-in 2. Exploration of museum objects in self-directed way and handled objects in room or focused on personal responses to objects. 3. Artmaking followed by verbal reflection	Facilitate exploration of self and connection with others through museum objects Create meaning-making opportunities using objects Emphasize concepts such as containment, metallization, transitional objects and space, attachment, and joint attention
Legari, personal communication, 2019 Hartman, 2019 (in press) Montreal Museum of Fine Art Autism Without Limits	Young adults with autism between the ages of 19–25 8–12 group members including volunteers	Three phases of 8-week sessions; 30-week initial program 1. Educational and free exploration gallery discussion about feelings and experiences. 2. Therapist integrates emojis and icons to discuss intensity of emotional experiences (Atwood protocol) 3. Discussions follow psychoeducation about a particular emotion. 4. The art therapist facilitates a studio artmaking session using the Expressive Therapies Continuum (ETC). The program provides lunch as a social component that enhances dynamic of group with art therapist	Promote socialization opportunities Enhance emotional awareness and expression Increase autonomy and decision-making

(Continued)

Table 2.2 (Continued)

Authors Museum, Program Title & Collaborating Partnerships	Population(s) Served	MBAT Program Structure and Protocol	Therapeutic Intentions
Coles & Harrison, 2018 Gloucester Folk Museum and City Museum and Art Gallery	Young adults ages 18–25 years with severe mental health issues 10 women	18-week art psychotherapy group focusing on themed boxes of museum objects 1. 15-minute introduction 2. 25-minute self-directed exploration of museum objects with art therapist 3. 30-minute artmaking session 4. 20-minute discussion	Enhance social inclusion and engagement Combat stigma about mental health Offer access to community resources
Reyhani Dejkameh & Shipps, 2019 Queens Museum ArtAccess Young Adult Programs Decade-long partnership with district 75 middle/high school classes	8–10 students with autism 15–21 Young adults with autism ages 17–25	Program 1: Special Arts Group that included gallery experience and weekly studio sessions including the culminating event and exhibition with other participating classes Program 2: Community-based platform hosted Open Art Studio bimonthly on Sundays	Increase awareness of vocational opportunities Improve quality of lives of families and individuals with autism Provided sense of community and diverse cultural understanding
M. Reyhani Dejkameh, personal communication, 2020 ArtAccess at Queens Museum and Queens College Special Inclusion Program	Young adults with ASD, ages 17–25	Program 3 with ArtAccess Grant funded multi-year museum internship initiatives 1. Hosted internships for students with autism as part of ArtAccess and later from Queens College Special Inclusion	Offer a space for socialization as young adults' transition from school to post-school life

| Salom, 2011 Archeological Museum in Bogotá, Museo Arqueologico Casa del Marques de San Jorge (in 2009) | 3–4 young adults | Applied Erikson's (1963) psychosocial developmental stages to therapeutic intentions 1. Gallery viewing of diverse collections. 20 minutes of view and sketch 2. Greeting and conversational time. Discussion on life choices and life stages 3. Artmaking with therapist includes drawings and clay sculptures, sharing and processing | Promote conversations about making life choices, resolving issues, interpersonal relationships, and the significance of work Explore universal symbols and healthy symbols of the self Explore personal identity |
| Alter-Muri, 1996 Museum gallery and museum trips as part of treatment planning | Male, 19 years, learning disability, psychosis, depression, and substance abuse Male mid-20s, developmental delay and behavioral challenges | 1. Viewed slides of artists from Cubism to outsider art 2. Discussed the lives of the artists 3. Created response artwork | Increase self-esteem, patience, development of identity, positive social interactions Help decrease stereotypical and repetitive imagery Decrease levels of frustration |

Shipps, 2019) and individuals with complex mental health challenges (Alter-Muri, 1996; Coles, Harrison, & Todd, 2019; Coles & Harrison, 2018).

The therapeutic intentions for young adult programs have emphasized identity development (Salom, 2011), socioemotional development and independence (Legari, personal communication, 2019), vocational goals and family support (Reyhani Dejkameh & Shipps, 2019), and mental health recovery (Coles et al., 2019; Coles & Harrison, 2018). The structure of three of the young adult programs follow longer-term interventions that span 18–20 weeks, respectively. The MMFA's program initially started as a 30-week program but was modified owing to need and appropriateness to host three phases of eight weekly sessions.

Within MBAT practice, many applications of theoretical approaches vary, including art psychotherapy, psychoeducation, open-studio, expressive therapies continuum (ETC), and psychosocial implications of Erikson's work (1963). It is also interesting to note that these programs have a global span, with programs in the Northeastern United States, Canada, England, Korea, and Colombia.

In addition to varying theoretical approaches, diverse collections and museum objects have been applied to explore therapeutic intentions. Some programs used museum objects aligning with local history and prehistory, natural history, decorative arts, and contemporary art (Coles et al., 2019) or Cubism and outsider art (Alter-Muri, 1996), whereas others followed careful selection of objects that related to personal emotional expression or symbols of the self. These objects were used to facilitate exploration of self and connection with others, create meaning-making opportunities, and explore personal responses.

Summary of Community-based Programs for Adult Groups

Community-based programs for diverse adult audiences across the life span host a variety of community partners with common efforts toward enriching the lives of diverse audiences. These initiatives seek to provide supportive and positive spaces for creative self-expression and socialization. The programs in the U.S. tend to emphasize open-studio workshops, often aligning well with accessibility programming in the museum. Programs in Europe tend to follow an art psychotherapy framework. The museums hosting these programs are diverse, ranging from a history museum's library and research center to the National Museum of Contemporary Art, in Athens. The programs offered here represent the diverse and broad scope of possibilities in museum access, education, art therapy, and wellness programming.

Creative Aging and Well-being

Creative aging programs typically seek to enhance emotional, cognitive, and physical health for older adults. Museums can positively contribute to the

Table 2.3 Community-based MBAT Programs for Diverse Adult Groups

Authors Museum, Program Title, & Collaborating Partnerships	Population(s) Served	MBAT Program Structure and Protocol	Therapeutic Intentions
Reyhani Dejkameh & Shipps, 2019 Queens Museum Please Touch 1983 Program and Open Studio Programs	Visually impaired persons (VIP) Individuals with diverse cognitive, emotional, intellectual, and physical abilities	Community-based art therapy with groups across the life span Weekend open studio for adults of various abilities from various community organizations 1. Storytelling and engagement with museum objects and collections 2. Artmaking focus is toward personal connections and open-ended questioning about the context of the museum objects	Enhance socialization and engagement in the community, social inclusion Provide sensory opportunities for individuals; offer different choices for empowerment Offer opportunities for self-expression and positive self-regard
Pantagoutsou, Ioannides, & Vaslamatzis, 2017 National Museum of Contemporary Art, Athens (EMST) with First Psychiatric Department of University of Athens, Eginition Hospital Greece	Adults ages 18 and old 10 participants motivated in art	Art psychotherapy, 12 weekly sessions for 2 hours over 3 months Emphasized conscious/unconscious projections, free association, and spontaneous expression 1. Viewed artwork through projections and slides 2. Discussed personal responses 3. During last two sessions, group reflected on work they had done over 10 sessions	Encourage self-expression, reflection, creativity, and critical thinking Explore self-image, insecurity, perception of control, gender identity and sexual orientation, roles in romantic and family relationships Provide corrective experiences, reflection

(Continued)

Table 2.3 (Continued)

Authors Museum, Program Title, & Collaborating Partnerships	Population(s) Served	MBAT Program Structure and Protocol	Therapeutic Intentions
Hamil, 2016 Art Therapy Access Program, Memphis Brooks Museum of Art Artworks grant from NEA	Several diverse audiences served VA centers Senior centers Juvenile detention centers Day centers	Access program designed to provide a supportive and creative environment 1. Multiple visits to the museum and museum tours for family/caregivers 2. Artmaking sessions with a registered art therapist 3. Resulting exhibition, Making Our Mark: A Creative Path for Change	Enhance dialogue and self-expression Enrich the lives of diverse communities Explore their personal narratives through artmaking and gallery discussions
Klorer, 2014 Missouri History Museum's Library and Research Center	270 participants in community workshops	1. Art therapist used historic documents and letters to chronicle local and family history 2. Sculptures and altered books were exhibited in the Missouri History Museum's library (2019) 3. Four community workshops were inspired, including 270 participants inquired into telling their own family stories through art	Explore family identity, generational influences and values, dynamics and relationships, and family of origin Preserve and pass down heritage to next generations

health and wellness of aging populations (Rosenblatt, 2014). One focus of these initiatives is to explore ways to increase the quality of life for individuals with cognitive decline, dementia, and Alzheimer's and their caregivers. Museum visits and discussions largely take place around personal reminiscence work while exploring memories, feelings, and associations to the artworks. The therapeutic intentions of these programs typically seek to decrease loneliness, increase social engagement, and reconnect with the self through exploring personal memories and experiences in a social and aesthetically inspiring setting.

A study by Camic, Baker, and Tischler (2016) used traditional and contemporary galleries to explore how art viewing in the gallery as well as artmaking activities over 8 weeks might improve the quality of life for 12 adults with mild-to-moderate dementia and their 12 caregivers. The study determined that these gallery-based art experiences provided intellectual stimulation, offered social opportunities for engagement, and created positive emotional experiences for the participants. The findings from this study inform and align well with several of the MBAT programs designed for similar aging populations. Table 2.4 outlines art therapy programs that align well with creative aging.

Summary of MBAT Programs that Emphasize Creative Aging

Many programs currently focus on aging adults with Alzheimer's and dementia and their caregivers. Several studies have explored the impact of artmaking and art viewing for both the aging adults and their caregivers. Additionally, programs have now begun to provide intellectually stimulating experiences in the museum. For instance, a new direction is in body positivity and focusing on contemporary works of artists who explore the personal responses to aging, self-esteem, attractiveness, or cultural standards of beauty (Wellcome Collection, 2020). There have been several museum exhibitions that have focused on body-positive content, as well as those that address agism through more contemporary works. These ideas, as well as a focus on reminiscence and life review, have been directions that art therapists have integrated into their work in the programs mentioned in this chapter.

MBAT Existing Programs Based on Presenting Issues and Needs

This section has focused on the MBAT programs that have been classified according to focus on specific age groups. The following tables will outline the existing MBAT programs that have been developed to address particular client issues such as complex mental health challenges, the cancer journey, immigration/acculturation issues, and mental health issues associated with the experience of traumatic events.

Table 2.4 MBAT Programs Emphasizing Creative Aging

Authors Museum, Program Title, & Collaborating Partnerships	Population(s) Served	MBAT Program Structure and Protocol	Therapeutic Intentions
Reyhani Dejkameh & Shipps, 2019 Art*Access* Queens Museum Creative Imagination Project	Individuals with dementia and Alzheimer's disease and caregivers Typically, aging LGBTQ+ older adults	Several museum-based art therapy sessions via therapeutic creative arts workshops that offer support and therapeutic experiences through creative arts engagement	Decrease isolation, stimulate cognitive ability, and increase quality of life (QOL)
Bennington et al., 2016 Blinded Museum in California	8 older adults from assisted-living facility in California reporting feelings of loneliness and wishing to make art	Phenomenological approach to exploring perspectives of older adults in group 1. Relaxed viewing tours in the museum focusing on four selected thematic paintings 2. Discussion about artworks focusing on reminiscence 3. Created response artwork in private space in the museum	Allow reminiscence work to take place Promote discussion about childhood experiences and memories Reflect themes such as hope, sorrow, and self-understanding, growth, appreciation, and social connection

Rosenblatt, 2014 The Creative Aging Program at The Phillips Collection, Senior Center and Wellness and Arts Center George Washington University Art Therapy Program	Groups of 10–15 individuals Older adults with memory loss, diabetes, stroke, Parkinson's disease, and other chronic illnesses and family members	Daily art therapy groups at the Wellness & Arts Center 1. Viewed museum digital archives and portraits together. Multi-visit program to the gallery using mindful looking, close looking, and inquiry discussions 2. 60-minute conversations about 3 artworks with groups of 10–15 members. Discussions focus on personal connections made with the themes in the galleries and artworks 3. Created self-portraits with the art therapist exploring life journeys and creative process Client artwork was presented at the Creative Ageing and Phillips Collection exhibition with 50 pieces created by 15 artwork response activities	Explore personal history and memory Provide empowerment through sense of accomplishment Foster activity, intellectual engagement, and social opportunities Cognitive and sensory stimulation, reducing stress, and connecting socially with peers
Salom, 2011 Museo Arqueologico Casa del Marques de San Jorge (Archaeological Museum in Bogotá) Fundación Voluntariado Juan Pablo II, care facility for older adults	10 older adults age 70 and older from a care facility and two nurses	Used psychosocial developmental stages (Erikson, 1963) to define therapeutic intentions for older adults. Used life-review approach to reflect on life experiences 1. 40-minute exploration of the environment, having tea and cookies, and conversational time 2. 15-minute viewing of a small exhibition that emphasized mirroring personal history with clay objects and themes that intersected between geography, history, culture, utility, and form 3. Artmaking session with watercolors painting, and painting experiences	Revisit histories and personal memories and share previous life experiences Promote social connection Explore personal feelings and memories Explore the self and lived experiences; reconnect with personal identity

Table 2.5 MBAT Programs for Individuals with Complex Mental Health Issues

Authors Museum, Program Title, & Collaborating Partnerships	Population(s) Served	MBAT Program Structure and Protocol	Therapeutic Intentions
Coles et al., 2019 Museum in the Park in Stroud (Gloucestershire)	Adults with complex mental health difficulties Groups included 6–10 participants	Two 12-week art psychotherapy groups 1. Check-in and self-directed exploration of museum objects from prehistory, natural history, decorative arts, and contemporary art 2. Object handling and discussion about responses to objects 3. Artmaking and verbal reflection	Objects facilitated exploration of self and connection with others Objects created meaning-making opportunities
Baddeley et al., 2017 Montreal Museum of Fine Arts (MMFA) and the Douglas Mental Health Institute Department	Eating disorders group of 12 or fewer each session	Art therapy groups held every 6 weeks: 1. Gallery visit follows discussion-based theme for 60–90 minutes focusing on 4–6 artworks/ objects 2. Explore abstract art/portraiture to emphasize therapeutic conversations central to eating disorders 3. Art therapy studio session to discuss emotions and the art therapy experience Included Creative Arts Therapies at Concordia University	Provided a supportive space for discussion about body image, beauty, and stereotypes Encouraged self-discovery and positive body image Promoted sense of belonging and community
Alter-Muri (1996) Various museum and galley visits	Inpatient and elderly individuals with chronic mental health and cognitive deficits	1. Visits to museum/gallery to explore client's preference and interest 2. Incorporated slides, art history context, and info about artists 3. Clients created artwork in response to these themes	Promoted reminiscence, self-acceptance with changes in life, and new identity Viewed artwork as source of inspiration

Summary of MBAT Programs for Individuals with
Complex Mental Health Issues

MBAT programs that have been designed for individuals with complex mental health issues have identified the value of viewing artwork as an inspiration and connection to personal lives. These protocols have incorporated this into treatment plans, such as described by Alter-Muri (1996), in addition to the creative expression of artmaking in session. The groups mentioned in these programs have structured their practices differently. Some groups took place over 4 weeks and others over 12 weeks. The session length ranges from 1 hour to 2.5 hours. They typically followed a group format that emphasizes a sense of belonging, community, and support. The MBAT therapeutic intention for issues related to complex mental health disorders varies. Some protocols have emphasized self-understanding, exploring one's meaning, or developing a creative identity in an effort to reframe and re-author one's narrative as it relates to mental health challenges. The museum is a space that offers the narrative concept as an easy venue to explore the personal narrative through artworks, museum objects, thematic exhibitions, and making personal connections to one's life.

A study by Colbert et al. (2013) explored how the personal narrative of adults experiencing psychosis and mental health issues may shift from one of stigma to self-understanding through participation in gallery-focused and reflective artmaking groups. This study took place at the Dulwich Picture Gallery in London and was in collaboration with the National Health Service (NHS). It used a protocol similar to art therapy programming that has been done: the gallery discussion focused on the context of the art in connection to the personal narratives of participants, and a 20-mintue gallery sketch and 30-minute individual narrative-focused artmaking session followed. Results from this study indicated that individuals with schizophrenia, bipolar, and schizoaffective disorders were able to reframe personal narratives associated with mental illness and develop a creative identity.

MBAT Program Opportunities for Health and Wellness

A more current direction museums have begun to embrace is the area of health, wellness, and improving the well-being of the public, rather than a focus on a particular visitor audience or client group. Several authors and researchers have explored how art museums may play a role in public health interventions (Camic & Chatterjee, 2013), as well as how they may benefit the lives of family members with relatives with mental health issues (Camic, Roberts, & Springham, 2011). For instance, the MMFA currently has developed programming with a wellness focus that complements the accessibility, educational, and art therapy structured programs the museum offers (Legari, personal communication, 2019). Wellness groups are starting to become an area of interest, and these models vary from incorporating mindfulness and contemplative experiences with artwork to engaging with art for the purpose of increasing creative expression and improving social connection in the community.

Table 2.6 MBAT Programs for Oncology Patients

Authors Museum, Program Title, & Collaborating Partnerships	Population(s) Served	MBAT Program Structure and Protocol	Therapeutic Intentions
Deane, Carman, & Fitch, 2000 McMichael Canadian Art Collection and Bayview Cancer Support Network, Kleinburg, Ontario	Cancer patients Groups of 10 or fewer	Session held for 2 hours weekly over 16 weeks using museum/ gallery in 100 acres of wilderness 1. Museum/ gallery viewing artwork that promotes reflection of thoughts and feelings 2. Opportunity to learn about artwork, focusing on artists' work that included landscapes, body image related to illness, self-portrait, and medical treatment reflections 3. Studio allowed free expression about the cancer journey Studio and gallery components viewed the art from phenomenological perspective, allowing participants to understand objective and subjective interpretation	Assist cancer patients to visually express their feelings about the cancer experience outside of the hospital Express and confront pain and feelings about body through imagery

The only program mentioned in the art therapy literature using MBAT was that of Deane, Carman, and Fitch (2000). However, various hospitals and museums currently support therapeutic programming using the arts for hospital patients. MBAT collaborations do exist in various medical settings and for patients with various health concerns. These programs often are mentioned on the hospital web pages or on the web page of the museum. There is a need for additional literature highlighting the benefits of such programs because there is a potential to benefit many patients and families facing challenging circumstances. The American Alliance of Museums (2013) noted the potential for art therapy to contribute to museum programming owing to the nature of the skill set of the art therapist who is able to offer work in groups, bedside artmaking, and electronic wellness programming. This has been noted as a direction museums can adopt so they may contribute toward health and wellness creative interventions within various medical settings.

Summary of MBAT Programs Emphasizing Immigration/ Acculturation/Cultural Identity

Owing to the international crisis of relocation and the need for societal and cultural interventions to help moderate the negative psychosocial effects related to acculturation and assimilation, art therapists have begun to use the museum as a space to offer healing and transformative experiences. These programs have emphasized the narratives of immigrants and refugees and seek to provide ways to tell stories and receive support from others, while reframing the dominant narrative and perception of immigrants and refugees to the public. One way of doing this has been to use client-led exhibitions in the museum to highlight the personal lived experience of Iranian and Syrian refugees through various expressive arts (Ioannides, 2016).

Salom (2015) presented another way of working with these issues by facilitating two art therapy groups for internally displaced indigenous women (IDIW) in Colombia of Wounaan and Guambiano ethnicities. These groups provided the opportunity for women to connect through conversations about gender issues, the role of women in the community, men's expectations, the skills needed to be a wife and a mother, independence, migration, and their hardships while using the visual narratives and the gallery artworks to explore cultural identity and other experiences related to their displacement. These programs explored diversity in thinking, backgrounds, and religious/social/ national/gender/sexual identity.

Summary of Exhibition Programs Promoting Awareness of Trauma

Peacock (2012) published a summary of museum education and art therapy collaborations mentioning these programs, referring to them as "exhibitions of historical events" and "museum exhibitions of therapeutic art," respectively.

Table 2.7 MBAT Programs Emphasizing Immigration/Acculturation/Cultural Identity

Authors Museum, Program Title, & Collaborating Partnerships	Population(s) Served	MBAT Program Structure and Protocol	Therapeutic Intentions
Ioannides, 2016 National Museum of Contemporary Art, Athens (EMST), and UN Refugee Agency	20 adult refugees from Syria and Iran	Narrative/ storytelling approach to interactive visual exhibition highlighting narrative stories of individuals who had been forced to leave homeland and were rebuilding lives in another country 1. Storytelling workshops for 2-hour long meetings held four times a week for 3 weeks 2. View 11 works belonging to the collection. Use photos and narratives to talk about daily life 3. Co-curated client exhibition Face Forward . . . Into My Home included translated personal narratives recorded on mp3 in various languages	Shared feelings, stories, associations, hopes, memories, and aspirations Discussed current situation and future goals Facilitated self-expression, promote social cohesion, and cultivate solidarity Communicate stressors associated with dislocation
Salom, 2015 Museo del Oro (Gold Museum) Bogotá, Colombia Sharing Stories with Images and Materials	Internally displaced indigenous women (IDIW) in Colombia of Wounaan and Guambiano ethnicities Wounaan group: 9 females ages 12–18 Guambiano group: 6 females ages 17–40	Community-based narrative studio approach 1. Cultural exchange through artistic exploration of materials and techniques. This took place at a semi-private workshop room suited to arts and crafts 2. Museum gallery visit. Participated in discussions about cultural traditions. Made connection to current experiences 3. Studio workshops (3 hours) included paper murals, clay sculptures, textile weaving, and materials unique to cultural heritage and traditions	Work through issues related to acculturation, loss, and adjustment Explore culture of origin and cultural identity Create visual narratives, tell personal stories; receive support from others with similar experiences

Table 2.8 MBAT Programs Using Client Exhibitions to Promote Awareness about Factors Associated with Trauma

Date of Program & Authors	Museum, Program Title & Collaborating Partnerships	Population(s) Served	Art Therapy Program Structure and Facilitation Style
Auslander & Thomashow, 2019	Michigan State University Museum	Survivors of sexual violence	Expressing narratives through expressive arts workshop. Trauma specialists, clinicians, and survivors co-curated exhibition Finding Our Voice: Sister Survivors Speak exhibition
Peacock (2012)	New Orleans Museum of Art	Children/families displaced owing to Hurricane Katrina	Expressing experiences of trauma, loss, anxiety, depression in individuals through artwork in exhibition Katrina Through the Eyes of Children: Art by Displaced Children at Renaissance Village
Gonzales-Dolginko, 2002	The Children's Museum of the Arts, New York City, NY	Children with history of acute trauma from 9/11	Groups met over 12 weekly sessions for 1–1.5 hours Expressed children's feelings about trauma from 9/11 as well as hopes for the future in Operation Healing: In the Shadow of Terror
Goodman & Henderson Fahnestock, 2002	Museum of City of New York and NYU Child Study Center	Artists ages 5–19 with PTSD and other mental health issues associated with trauma	Expression of feelings associated with 9/11 and raising awareness of PTSD symptoms in 80 pieces of artwork The Day Our World Changed: Children's Art of 9/11

The intentions of curating such exhibitions were to empower survivors who had been silenced to tell their stories through narratives, raise awareness of art therapy and trauma (from natural disasters, such as Hurricane Katrina), provide opportunities for self-expression, process emotions related to trauma, and raise awareness of PTSD symptoms and mental health (relating to natural disasters or collective trauma).

Programs listed in Table 2.8 outline some examples of co-curated client exhibitions with artwork created with an art therapist during workshops or group sessions. The art therapy program offered to diverse community populations provided a space to process emotions related to traumatic events. Exhibitions were designed to empower these individuals and to promote awareness to the public about mental health issues associated with traumatic events.

Summary of MBAT Programming

Museum-based art therapy programs are largely influenced by the scope and mission of the museum as well as the needs the program may have in curatorial or museum education departments. Thus, they fall typically within the accessibility programming framework or the museum education framework. Although some MBAT programs function more independently, others might include multiple collaborators and interdisciplinary team members contributing to the progress of one group or audience.

The Role of the Art Therapist within Interdisciplinary Programming

In most of the programming and services, art therapists work in an interdisciplinary context. Some art therapists work with an entire multidisciplinary team such as social workers, child life specialists, psychologists, or other clinical specialists, as well as museum staff such as curatorial staff, art historians, public program coordinators, museum educators, teaching artists, or docents. As well, sometimes art therapists work independently as co-leaders with a particular client group and focus on their work in a private setting without the collaborative aspect of the work.

Theoretical Orientation and Art Therapy Approaches

In general, MBAT programs are community-based in nature. Theoretical preferences include psychodynamic art therapy approaches, feminist theory, critical studies, phenomenological/existential approaches, group therapy, family therapy, narrative approaches, open-studio, or the ETC. When the term MBAT is described, the association and understanding of therapy vary and are broadly considered. Within the community-based model, the art therapist may facilitate the sessions and gallery experiences in different ways depending on the different therapeutic approaches being emphasized.

In humanistic approaches, including studio, narrative, phenomenological, or existential theories, there is an emphasis on the audience making personal meanings and connections to the object. In art psychotherapeutic frameworks, the facilitation style differs in that it promotes free association, exploration of the unconscious and conscious, and the experience of sublimation or catharsis through the artmaking process.

Collectively, MBAT protocols focus on the lived experiences and personal experiences of the individual in response to the artwork in the gallery. This narrative focus well suits a diverse client base and it allows variability in the strategies for interaction with museum objects and collections. It also relates well to a variety of methods of creative arts expression. A narrative focus can be applied to more structured, consistent groups and it can be facilitated in a 1-day workshop in a meaningful way. The MBAT protocols that have explored narratives allow people to express themselves, explore, reflect, and tell their own stories. The narrative approach may also focus on reframing or retelling a narrative to counter the dominant narrative (Colbert et al., 2013). In MBAT, there is potential for individuals to find their own voice, find meaning in life, and learn from hearing the stories of others.

Generally, the common framework being used in art therapy in European museums emphasizes art psychotherapy, looking at creative expression through spontaneous play, free association, and exploration of symbols and the unconscious (Coles et al., 2019; Coles & Harrison, 2018; Pantagoutsou, Ioannides, & Vaslamatzis, 2017), whereas a majority of the art therapy programs in the United States may not use the term "art therapy" as frequently in the titles of programs. This is impacted by the role of the art therapist working in the museum. Several of the recently published museum art therapy programs initiated by clinical art therapists working with the UK's NHS or other clinical setting have the objective of including museums or creating a bridge from their clinic to museums. These are not often programs that operate exclusively in the museum or are part of the actual museum structure, such as the Montreal Museum of Fine Arts (2020) or the Queens Museum of New York, which has its own art therapy program as part of the museum structure and funds a full-time art therapist.

In the United States, art therapists more often work independently with museums, and some art therapists are employed as staff within the museum or they participate in roles associated with grant-funded projects. These programs often tend to fall within the scope of accessibility programming or museum education programs. However, some art therapy groups may creatively move between these frameworks to accommodate and work with a particular client population, hosting structured groups that include a component of the museum as part of their creative interventions (Hartman, 2019; Treadon et al., 2006; Marxen, 2009). Art therapists who are employed in a museum typically understand the museum's dynamics and resources, as well as its collaborative team, more than a visiting clinical art therapist.

Some programs define their work in terms of creative expressive workshops or therapeutic arts workshops, rather than using the term "session" or "art therapy" or "art psychotherapy" (Canas, 2011). This language may differ depending on the scope and programming needs of the museum, the therapeutic intentions of the program, and the accessibility and inclusivity this language may suggest for different individuals who may associate stigma with the term "therapy."

Some programs are approached under a preventative, well-being, and wellness lens. These usually seek to enhance self-esteem, explore personal identity, promote healthy views toward oneself and others, increase tolerance for diverse perspectives, allow an outlet for self-expression, and meet the needs of diverse individuals (Canas, 2011). This focus aligns more with a community-based model than a clinical one.

Therapeutic Implications and Considerations in the Museum

Therapeutic implications for programming vary. They seek to promote relationships; enhance decision-making, communication, personal meaning, personal reflection, processing emotions through artwork, socialization opportunities, and community engagement; foster new identity, explore personal identity, and revisit parts of identity; aid self-discovery; and provide a creative outlet for self-expression and the chance to make connections between historical themes in objects, the context of artworks, and personal experiences.

Museum-based Art Therapy Session Structure

The structure and format for interacting and engaging with artworks in the gallery differ based on the program, needs and scope of the museum mission, and the style and approach of the art therapist collaborating in the program. In general, approaches to artmaking differ among the programs. Some programs offer sessions hosted outside the museum, including a final gallery tour and artmaking experience in the museum (Treadon et al., 2006). Other programs bring museum objects to community organizations off-site, such as medical or psychiatric hospitals or inpatient units (Deane et al., 2000; Reyhani Dejkameh & Shipps, 2019). Recently, art therapists have incorporated client-led exhibitions as part of the experience, hosting sessions in the museum gallery or inside private studio rooms near the gallery (Hartman, 2019; Coles & Harrison, 2018).

Conclusion

In addition to the programs mentioned in this chapter, research studies have documented results that may further influence MBAT practice. A study by

Betts et al. (2015) provided insight into how museum visitors experiencing exhibitions that focus on distressing content may use art therapy protocols to enhance empathy. According to Thomson et al. (2012), the act of handling tactile objects in addition to viewing museum objects promoted greater well-being improvements than only viewing or experiencing objects through touch. Implications from viewing artwork may be a cost-efficient way to offer psychosocial support to caregivers of family members with mental health issues (Camic et al., 2011). In the Dali Museum study of 176 children who improved in self-concept, researchers determined that participating in summer arts programming in the museum promoted both educational and therapeutic benefits (Kaufman et al., 2014). Finally, Klein's (2015) study highlighted opportunities for MBAT to accommodate and enhance the lives of veterans. These studies ultimately provide implications for art therapists who hope to expand the scope of practice in MBAT.

References

Alter-Muri, S. (1996). Dali to Beuys: Incorporating art history in art therapy treatment plans. *Art Therapy: Journal of the American Art Therapy Association, 13*(2), 102–107. http://dx.doi.org/10.1080/07421656.1996.10759203

American Alliance of Museums. (2013). Museums on call: How museums are addressing health Issues. Retrieved from: www.aam-us.org/wp-content/uploads/2018/01/museums-on-call.pdf

Auslander, M. & Thomashow, A. (2019). Sites of healing: The Michigan State University Museum turned to community co-curation to tell survivors' stories of sexual violence. *Museums, 35–40.* Retrieved from www.aam-us.org/2019/10/31/sites-of-healing-the-michigan-state-university-museum-turned-to-community-co-curation-to-tell-survivors-stories-of-sexual-violence/

Baddeley, G., Evans, L., Lajeunesse, M., & Legari, S. (2017). Body talk: Examining a collaborative multiple-visit program for visitors with eating disorders. *Journal of Museum Education, 42*(4), 345–353. https://doi.org/10.1080/10598650.2017.1379278

Bennington, R., Backos, A., Carolan, R., Etherington Reader, A., & Harrison, J. (2016). Art therapy in art museums: Promoting social connectedness and psychological well-being of older adults. *The Arts in Psychotherapy, 49,* 34–43. http://dx.doi.org/10.1016/j.aip.2016.013

Betts, D. J., Potash, J. S., Luke, J. J., & Kelso, M. (2015). An art therapy study of visitor reactions to the United States Holocaust Memorial Museum. *Museum Management & Curatorship, 30*(1), 21–43. https://doi.org/10.1080/09647775.2015.1008388

Camic, P. M., Baker, E. L., & Tischler, V. (2016). Theorizing how art gallery interventions impact people with dementia and their caregivers. *The Gerontologist, 56*(6), 1033–1041. https://doi.org/10.1093/geront/gnv063

Camic, P. M., & Chatterjee, H. J. (2013). Museums and art galleries as partners for public health. *Perspectives in Public Health, 133*(1), 66–71. https://doi.org/10.1177/1757913912468523

Camic, P. M., Roberts, S., & Springham, N. (2011) New roles for art galleries: Art-viewing as a community intervention for family carers of people with mental health problems. *Arts & Health, 3*(2), 146–159. https://doi.org/10.1080/17533015.2011.561360

Canas, E. (2011). Cultural institutions and community outreach: What can art therapy do? *Canadian Art Therapy Association Journal, 24*(2), 30–33. https://doi.org/10.1080/08322473.2011.11415549

Colbert, S., Cooke, A., Camic, P. M. & Springham, N. (2013) The art gallery as a resource for recovery for people who have experienced psychosis. *The Arts in Psychotherapy, 40*(2), 250–256. http://dx.doi.org/10.1016/j.aip.2013.03.003

Coles, A., & Harrison, F. (2018). Tapping into museums for art psychotherapy: An evaluation of a pilot group for young adults. *International Journal of Art Therapy, 23*(3), 115–124. https://doi.org/10.1080/17454832.2017.1380056

Coles, A., Harrison, F., & Todd, S. (2019). Flexing the frame: Therapist experiences of museum-based group art psychotherapy for adults with complex mental health difficulties. *International Journal of Art Therapy, 24*(2). https://doi.org/10.1080/17454832.2018.1564346

Deane, K., Carman, M. & Fitch, M. (2000). The cancer journey: Bridging art therapy and museum education. *Canadian Oncology Nursing Journal, 4*, 140. http://doi.org/10.5737/1181912x104140142

Erikson, E. H. (1963). *Youth: Change and challenge.* New York: Basic Books.

Gonzales-Dolginko, B. (2002). In the shadows of terror: A community neighboring the World Trade Center disaster uses art therapy to process trauma. *Art Therapy, 19*(3), 120–122. https://doi.org/10.1080/07421656.2002.10129408

Goodman, R. & Henderson Fahnestock, A. (Eds.) (2002). *The day our world changed: Children's art of 9/11.* New York: Harry N. Abrams.

Hartman, A. (2019). The museum as a space for therapeutic art experiences for adolescents with high functioning autism (HFA) [ProQuest Information & Learning]. In *Dissertation Abstracts International Section A: Humanities and Social Sciences, 80,* (2–A(E)).

Hamil, S. (2016). The art museum as a therapeutic space [Doctoral dissertation]. Graduate School of Arts and Social Science, Lesley University. Retrieved from: http://digitalcommons.lesley.edu/cgi/viewcontent.cgi?article=1036&context=expressive_dissertations

Ioannides, E. (2016). Museums as therapeutic environments and the contribution of art therapy. *Museum International, 68*(3–4), 98–109. https://doi.org/10.1111/muse.12125

Kaufman, R., Reinehardt, E., Hine, H., Wilkinson, B., Tush, P., Mead, B. & Fernandez, F. (2014). The effects of a museum art program on the self-concept of children. *Journal of the American Art Therapy Association, 31*(3), 118–125. https://doi.org/10.1080/07421656.2014.935592

Klein, D. L. (2015). The art of war: Examining museums' art therapy programs for military veterans. Retrieved from http://search.ebscohost.com/login.aspx?direct=true&AuthType=sso&db=ddu&AN=0BE05570FAC74B4B&site=eds-live

Klorer, G. (2014). My story, your story, our stories: A community art-based research project. *Art Therapy Journal of the American Art Therapy Association, 31*(4), 146–154. https://doi.org/10.1080/07421656.2015.963486

Linesch, D. (2004). Art therapy at the Museum of Tolerance: Responses to the life and work of Friedl Dicker-Brandeis. *The Arts in Psychotherapy, 31*, 57–66. https://doi.org/10.1016/j.aip.2004.02.004

Marxen, E. (2009). Therapeutic thinking in contemporary art: Or psychotherapy in the arts. *The Arts in Psychotherapy, 36*(3),131–139. https://doi.org/10.1016/j.aip.2008.10.004

Montreal Museum of Fine Arts. (2020). Art therapy. Retrieved from www.mbam.qc.ca/en/education-and-art-therapy/art-therapy/

Museum of Art and Archaeology at the University of Missouri, Columbia. (2019). *Community: Healing Arts Program.* Retrieved from https://maa.missouri.edu/education/community

Pantagoutsou, A., Ioannides, E. & Vaslamatzis, G. (2017) Exploring the museum's images – exploring my image (Exploration des images du musée, exploration de mon image). *Canadian Art Therapy Association Journal, 30*(2), 69–77. 10.1080/08322473.2017.1375769

Peacock, K. (2012). Museum education and art therapy: Exploring an innovative partnership. *Art Therapy: Journal of the American Art Therapy Association, 29*(3) 133–137. https://doi.org/10.1080/07421656.2012.701604

Reyhani Dejkameh, M. & Shipps, R. (2019). From please touch to Art*Access*: The expansion of a museum-based art therapy Program. *Art Therapy, 35*(4), 211–217. https://doi.org/10.1080/07421656.2018.1540821

Rosenblatt, B. (2014). Museum education and art therapy: Promoting wellness in older adults. *Journal of Museum Education, 39*(3), 293–301. doi.org/10.1080/10598650.2014.11510821

Salom, A. (2011). Reinventing the setting: Art therapy in museums. *Arts in Psychotherapy, 38*(2) 81–85. https://doi.org/10.1016/j.aip.2010.12.004

Salom, A. (2015). Weaving potential space and acculturation: Art therapy at the museum. *Journal of Applied Arts & Health, 6*(1), 47–62. https://doi.org/10.1386/jaah.6.1.47_1

Stiles, G. J. & Mermer-Welly, M. J. (1998). Children having children: Art therapy in a community-based early adolescent pregnancy program. *Art Therapy Journal of the American Art Therapy Association, 15*(3), 165–176. 10.1080/07421656.1989.10759319

Treadon, C. B. (2016). Bringing art therapy into museums. In D. E. Gussak & M. L. Rosal (Eds), *The Wiley handbook of art therapy* (487–497). Wiley Blackwell.

Treadon, C. B., Rosal, M. L., & Thompson Wylder, V. D. (2006). Opening the doors of art museums for therapeutic processes. *The Arts in Psychotherapy, 33*(4), 288–301. https://doi.org/10.1016/j.aip.2006.03.003

Thomson, L. M., Ander, E., Menon, U., Lanceley, A. & Chatterjee, H. (2012). Quantitative evidence for wellbeing benefits from a heritage-in-health intervention with hospital patients. *International Journal of Art Therapy: Inscape, 17*(2), 63–79. https://doi.org/10.1080/17454832.2012.687750

Wellcome Collection. (2020). *Exhibitions.* Retrieved from https://wellcomecollection.org/exhibitions

3 Creating a Community Partnership for Lasting Change

Museum Art Therapy with Juvenile Offenders

Paige Scheinberg and Kathy Dumlao

Introduction

Multidisciplinary professionals, such as art and museum educators and art therapists, and community members are persistently striving to help create personal, social, and cultural change and growth – often through art. This chapter will discuss how an art museum and an organization for juvenile offenders established and have continued to develop an impactful, long-term partnership through a group art therapy program.

The Museum as a Space for Art Therapy

Art therapy has been found in hospitals, psychiatric facilities, and schools for almost a century (Rubin, 2010). However, the use of the museum as a space for art therapy is relatively new. Treadon, Rosal, and Thompson Wylder (2006) provided an overview of the historical, cultural, and educational roles of the museum and museum educators to help art therapists better conceptualize the museum as a novel setting for art therapy. Peacock (2012) later reviewed and researched exhibits and therapeutic programs offered by art therapists and professionals in museums. This research illustrated the impact of and rich possibilities for these types of innovative partnerships. Recent articles have continued to explore the efficacy of art therapy in museums with diverse groups, including individuals who are blind or have low vision, individuals with autism, and those with diverse abilities (Reyhani Dejkameh & Shipps, 2019); adults with mental health difficulties (Coles, Harrison, & Todd, 2019; Coles & Harrison, 2018); older adults (Bennington et al., 2016; Rosenblatt, 2014); individuals with dementia and their caregivers (Camic, Tischler, & Pearman, 2014; Camic, Baker, & Tischler, 2016; Reyhani Dejkameh & Shipps, 2019); individuals with eating disorders (Thaler et al., 2017); and displaced indigenous women (Salom, 2015).

The impact and power of the arts for healing and transformation with at-risk and justice-involved youth have been well documented (Gardner, Hager, & Hillman, 2018; OJJDP, 2016). As a result, community settings, such as museums, are increasingly exploring and stepping into their role to help facilitate

DOI: 10.4324/9781003014386-3

and create spaces for social, cultural, and personal change (Anderson, 2012; King, 2018; Silverman, 2010). Research and publications on art therapy with juvenile and adult offenders have primarily examined working with inmates and those in inpatient mental health settings (Gussak, 1997, 2004, 2006, 2007, 2009, 2020; Hartz & Thick, 2005; Kõiv & Kaudne, 2015; Larose, 1987; Persons, 2009). These studies have found art therapy to have several benefits, including enhancing self-image and self-esteem; improving mood and locus of control; and reducing challenging behaviors. However, there were no previous examples found of art therapists working with juvenile offenders in a museum setting.

Memphis Brooks Museum of Art

Located at the heart of Memphis, Tennessee, the Memphis Brooks Museum of Art is the oldest fine arts museum in the state and one of the largest art museums in the American South. The mission of the museum is "to enrich the lives of our diverse community through the museum's expanding collection, varied exhibitions, and dynamic programs that reflect the art of world cultures from antiquity to the present" (Brooks Museum, 2020, np). The Brooks Museum houses the only collection of world art in a three-state region, featuring more than 10,000 works of art that were made over the course of 5,000 years. Through more than a century of service to the Mid-South, the Brooks Museum continues to fulfill the purpose of its founder, Bessie Vance Brooks, as a "repository, conservatory, and museum of art . . . for the enjoyment, inspiration, and instruction of our people" (Memphis Brooks Museum of Art, 2004, p. 10).

The Brooks Museum's Art Therapy Access Program (ATAP) is a clear reflection of the museum's values and dedication to transforming lives through the power of art. At the program's core is the belief that art and art therapy have the power to inspire and encourage self-expression and to transform lives by providing new ways of seeing and expressing oneself. The art therapy program helps ensure that the museum is accessible to people across the life span with varying needs, including those who may not otherwise see or typically find themselves in an art museum. Likewise, the museum's commitment to inclusion and diversity is reflected in the program's outreach to underserved communities and mindfulness of financial accessibility to partners and participants. In addition, the ATAP is implemented utilizing best practices, such as working with a credentialed art therapist, promoting adherence to confidentiality, and striving to improve through evaluation, communication, and adjusting the program's offerings as needed.

Brooks Museum's Art Therapy Access Program

The Brooks Museum's Education Department began the ATAP in 2007, partnering with a local organization that provides support for people with Alzheimer's and their caregivers (Peacock, 2012). This program (and similar partnerships that followed) primarily occurred offsite at partner locations. These partnerships were dependent on grant funding, which limited them to pilot programs, making it difficult to build ongoing relationships with partners, provide continuity of services to partners and the community, maintain regular work with our (contract) art therapist, and ensure the longevity of the ATAP.

In 2015, the museum's director of education and art therapist (the authors of this article) began reimagining the goals and structure of the ATAP in an effort to increase community impact, better utilize the unique environment of the museum, and ensure the program's sustainability. One driving change was to facilitate art therapy programs at the museum, which required ongoing discussions about how to adapt art therapy most effectively to museum protocols and adapt the museum to the needs of art therapy groups. Considerations included creating art in the galleries and scheduling needs and potential conflicts. Further essential changes included making a financial commitment to the ATAP by including programming in the museum budget, expanding art therapy educational and advocacy offerings, and searching for partner organizations with shared long-term interests and values.

Creating a New Long-term Partnership: Juvenile Intervention and Faith-based Follow-up (JIFF)

After defining these changes for the future of the ATAP, Juvenile Intervention and Faith-based Follow-up (JIFF) emerged as our first long-term partner in late 2015. JIFF is a local nonprofit for male youth who have been referred by the juvenile court system. Through mentorship and a small-group, classroom-based approach, JIFF programs place an emphasis on the *Six Hs* – head, heart, health, home, hire-ability, and hobbies in order to reduce recidivism, facilitate effective reentry, and help the youth plan for the future.

Building the Partnership

Building any new partnership takes time, including the need to develop trust and rapport between partners (Mattessich & Monsey, 2001). This was especially important for this partnership because JIFF staff and youth were not familiar with art therapy, nor were they regular museumgoers. In an effort to help JIFF leaders become more familiar with art therapy and how it could benefit their youth, ATAP staff shared art therapy resources and described how the museum can serve as a safe, inspiring, exploratory setting for art therapy.

Another focal point was to address JIFF leaders' concerns about potential cultural challenges surrounding the stigma of mental health and therapy. For example, JIFF leaders requested to explore alternative names for the program owing to apprehension about possible negative perceptions by the youth, guardians, and staff about "therapy." The art therapist agreed that the youth needed to be asked what they would like to call the group. Yet, she emphasized the importance of transparency and honesty to not only let the youth participants know she was a mental health professional, but also how art and the art therapy group could help them discover, grow, heal, share, and create change in themselves and their lives. Over the years, the youth have chosen to refer to their groups as "art therapy" and have expressed pride about their experiences and accomplishments within the unique opportunity of being in the art therapy program.

Preparing for the Pilot Program

Many logistical details also needed to be addressed to launch the January 2017 pilot art therapy program. These included:

- Identifying the goals of the art therapy partnership
- Defining the roles and responsibilities of each partner organization
- Scheduling the sessions (i.e., length, frequency, duration, days, times)
- Deciding upon the number of youths in the group
- Creating and collecting art therapy consent forms
- Planning transportation
- Finalizing museum after-hours logistics (due to JIFF program hours)

Roles and Responsibilities of the Partners

This art therapy program is a true partnership, as it depends upon and is strengthened by the multidisciplinary nature, abilities, and experiences of its leaders. Each person and organization has an essential and ongoing role in developing, executing, and strengthening the partnership.

- *The art therapist*: Works closely with the museum's director of education to plan and develop the partnership and programs. Provides research and development information for the museum and the partner to better understand the efficacy and potential impact of art therapy. Creates and edits art therapy consent forms. Advises on budget and costs. Establishes and evaluates progress of group goals and needs throughout each program. Primarily plans each art therapy session (i.e., theme, goals, art viewing, directive, and materials). Leads partnership program meetings.
- *The museum's director of education*: Works closely with the art therapist to plan and develop the partnership and programs. Confirms budgetary and logistical requirements for running the groups at the museum. Attends meetings. Depending on availability, museum professionals' roles and responsibilities may vary. For example, the director of education may take the lead in helping develop and plan each partnership, while another museum education staff (or specially trained docent) may help co-lead and plan the groups. For this partnership, the director of education has also been the museum educator throughout all sessions.
- *The partner/JIFF*: Selects the mentor and group of young men who will participate. Collects consent forms from each participant and guardian.

Provides transportation to the museum for each session. Attends planning, kick-off, mid-program, and debrief meetings. Communicates changes in scheduling, participants, needs, and so on (as required). Partner staff include: executive director, program director, mentor director, and mentor/s.

Considerations

After implementing two art therapy programs with JIFF per year since the pilot, we have learned regular meetings are vital to the health and success of the partnership. For example, each program begins with a kick-off meeting with JIFF leadership and the group mentor. During kick-off meetings, we discuss art therapy, group goals, and consent forms; explain the flow of the sessions; define roles; and answer questions. A mid-program meeting allows ATAP leaders and the JIFF mentor to assess progress and explore solutions to any challenges. Finally, a debrief meeting is held with the JIFF mentor and leaders to review the program outcomes and begin planning for the next program. These meetings keep the partnership on track and communication open, while also providing opportunities to share feedback, clarify roles, discuss challenges and solutions, and continue to look for ways to improve.

Art Therapy Program Overview

Program Structure

JIFF's 16-week program for teenage male youth with an average of three or more arrests (some aggravated offenses) was chosen for the ATAP partnership. This program has a full after-school schedule with distinct requirements and objectives; thus, we needed to ensure the art therapy group aligned with its current goals, objectives, and needs.

After reviewing schedules and goals, we decided on six, weekly 2-hour sessions with a maximum of ten youth for the pilot art therapy group. The partners believed this would provide adequate time to establish group dynamics and achieve the program goals (detailed in the following section). In addition, JIFF's 16-week program had open, rolling enrollment, so we hoped this length of time would allow for a meaningful experience, whether the youth attended one or all sessions.

Each partner knew trial and error would be needed to build an effective and successful art therapy program. After almost 5 years of continuous JIFF art therapy partnerships, some structural components have remained constant, while others are flexible as we continue to explore what works best for the group and needs of both partners. Upon the completion of the pilot program, the art therapist advocated to increase the number of sessions to eight, owing to observing and feeling that the group termination was premature for most group members. Since then, all art therapy groups have included eight sessions (varying from 6 to 8 weeks), which has had positive outcomes.

Considerations

JIFF's program structure has changed from open enrollment to set cohorts, and, as a result, group attendance and participants are more consistent. The new cohort structure appears to support enhanced vulnerability and heightened authenticity in the creative processes, artwork, and discussions. Furthermore, we have observed more meaningful group dynamics when working with a cohort who is further into the JIFF program (compared with newly formed cohort groups), possibly owing to preexisting group rapport and trust, as well as greater investment in each other, the group experience, and their time at JIFF.

Program Goals and Approaches

The therapeutic goals of the JIFF art therapy groups are guided by the Positive Psychology PERMA model: positive emotions; engagement and flow; positive relationships; meaning and purpose; and achievement and mastery (Seligman, 2011; Wilkinson & Chilton, 2018). Together with JIFF's Six Hs, these models effectively help youth participants better understand their emotions, relationships, strengths, goals, and hopes for their life. Furthermore, by encouraging each group member to share their goals and needs each session, their sense of ownership, investment, and engagement in the program persists.

To achieve the program goals, we invite the use of multiple modes of self-expression, including verbalizations, viewing and creating art, music, movement, and writing. Informed by the expressive therapies continuum (Hinz, 2009), a variety of studio art materials – that is, for drawing, painting, sculpture, mixed media – are utilized throughout the studio experientials to meet the youth where they are emotionally, developmentally, and artistically. This also allows participants to explore and experience a range of artistic and therapeutic processes and directives.

Session Structure

Each JIFF art therapy session occurs at the Brooks Museum and has a similar structure:

1. Arrive and gather – greet JIFF group members and mentor
2. Creative warm-up – create a scribble drawing in a gallery
3. Explore and discuss – focus on a goal or theme through a piece of art or collection
4. Create and discuss – engage in an art experiential and group discussions in the art studio
5. Depart – escort participants outside

Sessions last between 1.5 and 2 hours, with the gallery and studio times fluctuating, depending on the respective goals, themes, and needs of the current group and session.

Considerations

Arrange stools or chairs in a circle in the gallery for the group to gather and settle into the session. Provide boards for drawing on laps, medium-sized paper, and colored pencils (only pencils are allowed in the galleries, owing to museum protocol) for the scribble drawing. Artworks are kept in a secured location at the museum throughout the art therapy program to ensure group members can view their pieces during the final group session, as well as participate in any potential exhibits.

Multidisciplinary Roles in the Art Therapy Sessions

The most effective, appropriate roles and responsibilities of the multidisciplinary professionals helping facilitate each art therapy session have developed over time and with collaborative discussions and observations. It is vital to discuss the roles of each session leader during the kick-off meeting before each program starts, so that the leaders are unified and have clarity and direction for their roles and expectations. Table 3.1 summarizes leader roles and engagement throughout each art therapy session from preparation to conclusion.

Table 3.1 Multidisciplinary Roles in Museum Art Therapy Sessions

	Art Therapist	Museum Educator	Program Mentor
Planning: themes & goals	✓*	✓	(✓)
Planning: gallery component	✓*	✓*	
Planning: studio (art process)	✓*	(✓)	
Arrival/departure	✓	✓	✓
Scribble drawing: guide	✓*		
Scribble drawing: create	(✓)	✓	✓
Scribble drawing: group discussion	✓*	✓	✓
Gallery discussions: art & history	✓	✓*	
Gallery discussions: relate to self & goals	✓*	(✓)	(✓)
Studio process: guide art directive	✓*	(✓)	
Studio process: create art	(✓)	(✓)	✓
Studio process: group discussion	✓*	✓	✓
Behavioral challenges	✓*	✓	✓

Notes: ✓* = primary role; ✓ = participates; (✓) = sometimes participates.

Sample Eight-session Art Therapy Group

After running multiple art therapy group programs with JIFF, we have discovered an array of museum pieces and group topics, themes, and art directives that resonate with many of our participants. The following is an example of eight art therapy sessions we facilitated with JIFF youth. As you will read, the sessions were guided by the needs and requests of the group members. The overarching goals stay the same with each new group, allowing some sessions to be replicated; however, the artworks viewed in the galleries and the art therapy directives and materials used in the studio often change to meet individual needs and requests.

Sessions 1–8: Warming Up and Assessing Participants

At the start of each art therapy session, group members were led through a brief "scribble drawing" and reflective discussions in a museum gallery (Figure 3.1). This warm-up drawing became a ritual that helped participants relax, transition into the group, and establish a safe space and creative practice for self-expression. In addition, group members progressively learned and practiced how to ask questions about art, talk about their creations, and notice patterns or themes as they arose in the art, questions, and reflections (as a group or individually).

As a foundational art therapy assessment (Cane, 1951; Winnicott, 1971), the art therapist also used verbalizations and observations during and after the creation of group members' scribble drawings – that is, mood, affect, focus, investment, use of the materials, graphic indicators, and symbolism – to quickly assess mental and emotional states and presenting personal strengths for each participant in each session. This form of assessment has been particularly helpful when group attendance and participants have fluctuated.

Discussion

Over the years, many participants have shown an interest in taking on leadership roles in the group. For example, a group member may lead the scribble drawing with assistance from the art therapist (as needed). Some group members have requested to lead this directive, or group members or leaders may encourage others to lead. Members and leaders have noted and observed increased engagement, confidence, and group investment after leading this aspect of the group.

Session 1: Identifying Expectations and Setting Goals

During the first session, the group explored most of the museum galleries and exhibitions to help participants feel more comfortable in the museum setting, identify their preferences in art, and cultivate curiosity for further explorations.

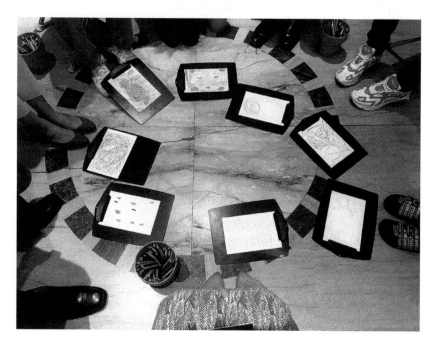

Figure 3.1 Group members and leaders create and discuss their scribble drawings at the
          beginning of each art therapy session

Photo Credit: Paige Scheinberg

Later, group members created a group poster that identified and listed guidelines, goals, expectations, hopes, and a name for their group.

Discussion

We often see many of the young men "come alive" during their time exploring
the entirety of the museum. Many participants have never been to a museum,
so this can be an empowering and inspiring experience. With the incredibly
diverse collection at the Brooks come many options and possibilities for connecting with art, subject matter, genres, and materials.

  The group guidelines poster is treated as a "living" document that can be
referenced and added to at any time. Poster items often include behavioral
and interpersonal guidelines (i.e., respect and confidentiality), exploring and
expressing thoughts and emotions, and art to view and create. The poster can
also be helpful for established group members to utilize when welcoming and
orienting new members. For example, group members refer to their poster to
explain the goals and expectations they have created for the group and ask if
the new member has anything he would like to add. Group leaders also call

attention to the poster when the group or individuals need to refocus or exhibit a behavior that does not align with their expectations and group goals.

Sessions 2–3: Telling Stories and Expressing Emotion

At the end of the first session, group members requested to learn more about art by first creating their own stories about the art on view, and then by hearing more about the history and artists from group leaders. During the following sessions, group members selected collection pieces to imagine and share stories about with the group. After sharing their stories, group members were encouraged to ask questions and add to each other's stories by exploring artistic choices, emotions, relationships, history, and culture. In the studio, group members were asked to "Create a piece of art that tells a story about your life" and, later, "Create a piece of art expressing an emotion we discovered or experienced in the galleries." Drawing and painting materials were offered for the participants to choose from.

Sample Brooks Museum pieces used were:

* *The Hen and the Hawk* (1934, oil on canvas), John Steuart Curry (1897–1946)
* *The Engineer's Dream* (1931, oil on panel), Thomas Hart Benton (1889–1975)

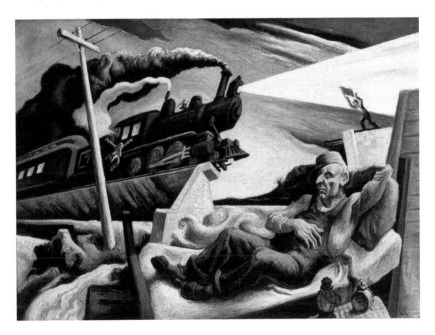

Figure 3.2 Thomas Hart Benton, *The Engineer's Dream*, 1931

Discussion

Emotional vocabulary and knowledge of artistic approaches and techniques have varied significantly with each group member, so it is important for the group leaders to be mindful of the language and terminology used during discussions. The museum educator and art therapist frequently ask questions to inspire discussions about the artists' materials, choices, and techniques, while the art therapist primarily facilitates group discussions identifying pieces in the collection that express or evoke an emotion, defining emotions, and sharing emotional experiences.

Session 4: Discovering Strengths

At this point in the group experience, group leaders and group members noticed and identified personal strengths. Using the VIA Classification of Character Strengths and Virtues (Peterson & Seligman, 2004), group members were led through a group discussion about the 24 character strengths. As each strength was discussed, individuals were asked to identify current perceived personal strengths and strengths they would like to cultivate. Then, group members were asked to locate an animal from collection pieces that related to or represented their top strengths. Guided by gallery discoveries and discussions about strengths and abilities, the youth used model magic in the art studio to "Create a sculpture of an animal that closely relates to your strengths and personality. The animal can be real or imagined and inspired from the museum collection or elsewhere" (Figure 3.3).

Sample Brooks Museum pieces used were:

- *Bull* (1st century B.C.E.–2nd century C.E., bronze), unknown maker
- *Torso of Pan* (1st century B.C.E.–1st century C.E., marble), unknown artist

Discussion

Exploring and establishing a language and listing personal strengths for each group member have proved to be effective, empowering, and inspiring components. Throughout the remainder of the group sessions, character strengths are explored, discussed, and encouraged in a number of ways, including reflecting (questioning and examining strengths in oneself – past, present, and future), strengths-spotting (noticing strengths in others), taking action (purposefully utilizing strengths in daily life), and finding balance (being mindful of over- or underuse of one's strengths; Niemiec & McGrath, 2019).

Sessions 5–6: Exploring Parts of Self

Portraits throughout the museum collection were selected to further examine identity, strengths, and personas. Discussions included, (1.) what the artist wants and allows you to see and know about the subject or self through the

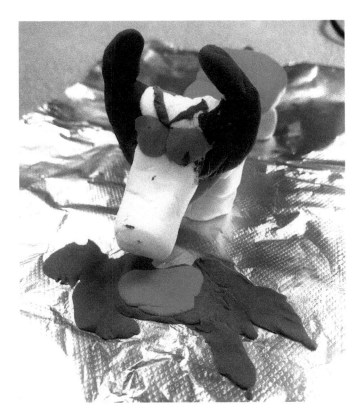

Figure 3.3 JIFF participant's sculpture of an animal to represent his personal strengths

Photo Credit: Paige Scheinberg

composition, materials, and title; and (2.) what we believe we know about the person based on our own observations, feelings, and experiences. In the studio, group members created an "inside/outside mask." On the front (outside) of the mask, participants were asked to "Create about the strengths and aspects of your personality that you typically or more easily allow people to see and know about you." On the back (inside) of the mask, group members were asked to "depict personal strengths, thoughts, and feelings that are often more challenging to express or share with others" (see Figure 3.5). Various drawing and painting materials were offered, and individuals were encouraged to work abstractly and/or realistically.

Discussion

We have found that group members typically request and require a considerable amount of time in the studio to create their masks, as compared with previous studio processes and directives. In addition, the youth consistently express

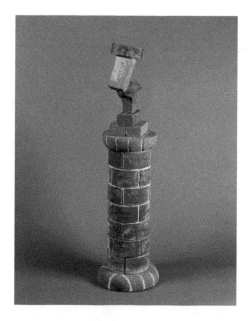

Figure 3.4 Robert Arneson, *Brick Self-Portrait*, 1979–81

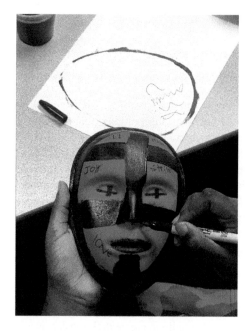

Figure 3.5 JIFF youth creating his "inside/outside" mask

Photo Credit: Paige Scheinberg

and exhibit increased investment, honesty, personal aesthetic and symbolism, and vulnerability as they create, finalize, and share their masks.

Sample Brooks Museum pieces used were:

- *Brick Self-Portrait* (1981, ceramic), Robert Arneson (1930–92)
- *Obscure Delites* (1983, acrylic, masonite, wood), Jim Nutt (1938–)

Sessions 7–8: Establishing Future Goals and Hopes

While viewing *Drawing Memory: Essence of Memphis* (2017), a mural by Victor Ekpuk (born 1964), group members identified and discussed personal and cultural symbolism that appeared to tell stories of their city's history and related to their current lives, communities, and the world around them. As a result, the group was inspired to create a final collaborative piece that allowed group members to illustrate and affirm their future goals and hopes for themselves and their communities, as well as leave a legacy for future JIFF participants. (Figure 3.7.) The final piece – a large mixed-media canvas – can be viewed on display at JIFF.

Discussion

During the final session, the art therapist and museum educator organize and display group member artwork in a "mini exhibit." This experience invites group members to observe, appreciate, reflect upon, and further explore the meaning of their pieces – individually and as a series or collection.

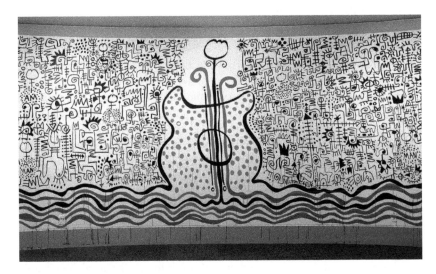

Figure 3.6 Victor Ekpuk (Nigerian American, b. 1964), *Drawing Memory of Memphis*, Acrylic paint on wall

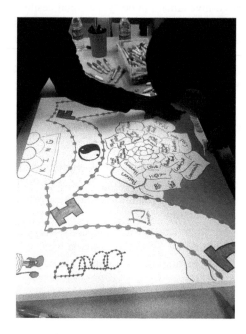

Figure 3.7 JIFF group members complete their final piece about their future goals and hopes for themselves and their communities, as well as to leaving a legacy for future JIFF participants

Photo credit: Paige Scheinberg

Art Therapy Exhibitions

We have successfully organized two JIFF art therapy exhibitions and private receptions. (Figure 3.8.) Organizing these 3–4-month exhibitions in the museum's education gallery depends on several factors, including: alignment with group goals and needs, participant desire and consent to participate, ample artwork to display, and museum gallery scheduling and availability. The art therapist primarily curates the exhibition, with the support and assistance of the museum's director of education (and/or museum educator) and museum installation staff.

Overall, we have found these exhibitions to support our goals and not only enhance the participant experience of art therapy, but also energize and ignite curiosity, creativity, and self-expression in other JIFF youth and staff who come to see the exhibition. One past participant described his pride, sense of accomplishment, and life-changing experience in art therapy as he viewed his artwork hung in his group's exhibition, stating

> Art be helping me get through life because of y'all. . . . It feels good. . . . I ain't never did nothing good enough for it to get displayed. I've barely even walked across stages in my life. So, it felt good to see something that I did – me and other troubled kids did – to get put up on a wall to be seen by a lot of people.

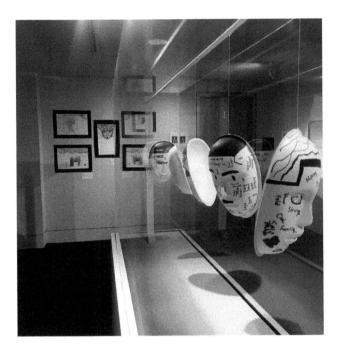

Figure 3.8 2017–18 JIFF art therapy exhibit at the Brooks Museum. *Making Our Mark: A Creative Path for Change*

Photo credit: Paige Scheinberg

It is not only the lives of the JIFF youth that are changed and enriched through the art therapy program and resulting exhibitions. Our visitors and community members gain new perspectives and empathy for the complex lives of these young men. When viewing their artwork, museum visitors could see the young men's stories, strengths, emotions, authenticity, and resilience – often challenging assumptions about and biases towards youth offenders. In addition, the public gains increased knowledge and understanding of the benefits and impact of art therapy.

Outcomes and Considerations

> Youth who typically are not encouraged or appreciated found that art [therapy] gave them a form of expressing their feelings and gave them a greater sense of self-worth. . . . What often takes weeks to peel back the layers of their issues and who you are really working with is accelerated through art therapy.
>
> (Richard Graham, executive director of JIFF)

Our experiences with the JIFF art therapy groups have emphasized there will never be a group art therapy "formula" that works for all our JIFF participants, but, if we remain flexible, open, and creative, we will find ways to meaningfully connect with each young man. In the final session of each group, group members and the JIFF mentor are asked to complete a brief evaluation form that measures personal, artistic, and emotional changes and reflections. Almost all evaluations have reported an "Excellent" experience, growth, and improvements in the topics noted above, and a positive recommendation of the program to others. To support and encourage their newfound connection to creative expression and personal growth through art, all group members who complete the program are given a bag with art materials and museum passes.

As we prepare for upcoming JIFF partnerships, we are adapting our program to offer a pilot telehealth group art therapy program (owing to the current COVID-19 pandemic). We are also exploring additional pre- and post-program mental health assessments and evaluations that could allow program staff to better understand potential needs of the youth and impacts of the art therapy group.

The art therapy partnership between the Brooks Museum and JIFF started in 2015, with a year and a half of building and planning, and has flourished into a dedicated, collaborative relationship between two community organizations that have developed impactful, innovative art therapy experiences. The time and financial commitments made by the Brooks Museum and JIFF have resulted in a unique, wholehearted investment, which allows for and encourages reflection and improvement on an ongoing basis. Both partners remain committed to growing and learning with each group and young man that participate in the art therapy partnership program.

References

Anderson, G. (Ed.) (2012). *Reinventing the museum: The evolving conversation of the paradigm shift.* New York: Altamira Press.

Bennington, R., Backos, A., Harrison, J., Etherington, A. & Carolan, R. (2016). Art therapy in art museums: Promoting social connectedness and psychological well-being of older adults. *The Arts in Psychotherapy, 49,* 34–43.

Brooks Museum. (2020, September 18). Mission and vision. Retrieved from: www.brooksmuseum.org/about

Camic, P. M., Baker, E. L., & Tischler, V. (2016). Theorizing how art gallery interventions impact people with dementia and their caregivers. *The Gerontologist, 56*(6), 1033–1041.

Camic, P. M., Tischler, V. & Pearman, C. H. (2014). Viewing and making art together: A multi-session art-gallery-based intervention for people with dementia and their carers. *Aging and Mental Health, 18*(2), 161–168.

Cane, F. (1951). *The artist in each of us.* London: Thames & Hudson.

Coles, A. & Harrison, F. (2018). Tapping into museums for art psychotherapy: An evaluation of a pilot group for young adults. *International Journal of Art Therapy, 23*(3), 115–124. DOI:10.1080/17454832.2017.1380056

Coles, A., Harrison, F. & Todd, S. (2019). Flexing the frame: Therapist experiences of museum-based group art psychotherapy for adults with complex mental health difficulties. *International Journal of Art Therapy, 24*(2), 56–67. DOI:10.1080/174548 32.2018.1564346

Gardner, A., Hager, L. L. & Hillman, G. (2018). *Prison arts resource project: An annotated bibliography.* Art Works, National Endowment for the Arts. Retrieved from: www.americansforthearts.org/node/100823

Gussak, D. (1997). Breaking through barriers: Advantages of art therapy in prisons. In D. Gussak & E. Virshup (Eds.), *Drawing time: Art therapy in prisons and other correctional settings* (1–11). Chicago: Magnolia Street.

Gussak, D. (2004). A pilot research study on the efficacy of art therapy with prison inmates. *The Arts in Psychotherapy, 31*(4), 245–259.

Gussak, D. (2006). The effects of art therapy with prison inmates: A follow-up study. *The Arts in Psychotherapy, 33,* 188–198.

Gussak, D. (2007). The effectiveness of art therapy in reducing depression in prison populations. *International Journal of Offender Therapy and Comparative Criminology, 5*(4), 444–460.

Gussak, D. (2009). The effects of art therapy on male and female inmates: Advancing the research base. *The Arts in Psychotherapy, 36,* 5–12.

Gussak, D. E. (2020). *Art and art therapy with the imprisoned: Recreating identity.* New York: Routledge.

Hartz, L. & Thick, L. (2005). Art therapy strategies to raise self-esteem in female juvenile offenders: A comparison of art psychotherapy and art as therapy approaches. *Art Therapy, 22,* 70–80.

Hinz, L. D. (2009). *Expressive therapies continuum: A framework for using art in therapy.* New York: Routledge.

King, L. (2018). *Art therapy and art museums: Recommendations for collaboration.* (Unpublished master's thesis). Indiana University, Indianapolis, IN.

Kõiv, K. & Kaudne, L. (2015). Impact of integrated arts therapy: An intervention program for young female offenders in correctional institution. *Psychology, 6,* 1–9. http://dx.doi.org/10.4236/psych.2015.61001

Larose, M. E. (1987). The use of art therapy with juvenile delinquents to enhance self-image, *Art Therapy, 4*(3), 99–104. DOI:10.1080/07421656.1987.10758708

Mattessich, P. & Monsey, B. (2001). *Collaboration: What makes it work. A review of research literature on factors influencing successful collaboration* (2nd ed.). Saint Paul, MN: Amherst H. Wilder Foundation.

Memphis Brooks Museum of Art. (2004). *Collection highlights from the Memphis Brooks Museum of Art.* Memphis, TN: Memphis Brooks Museum of Art.

Niemiec, R. M. & McGrath, R. E. (2019). *The power of character strengths: Appreciate and ignite your positive personality.* Cincinnati, OH: VIA Institute on Character.

Office of Juvenile Justice and Delinquency Prevention (OJJDP). (2016). Literature review: Arts-based programs and arts therapies for at-risk, justice-involved, and traumatized youths. Retrieved from: www.ojjdp.gov/mpg/litreviews/Arts-Based-Programs-for-Youth.pdf

Peacock, K. (2012). Museum education and art therapy: Exploring an innovative partnership. *Art Therapy: Journal of the American Art Therapy Association, 29*(3), 133–137. DOI:10.1080/07421656.2012.701604

Persons, R. W. (2009). Art therapy with serious juvenile offenders: A phenomenological analysis. *International Journal of Offender Therapy and Comparative Criminology, 54,* 433–453.

Peterson, C. & Seligman, M. (2004). *Character strengths and virtues: A handbook and classification.* New York: Oxford University Press.

Reyhani Dejkameh, M. & Shipps, R. (2019). From please touch to Art*Access*: The expansion of a museum-based art therapy program, *Art Therapy*, *35*(4), 211–217. DOI:10.1080/07421656.2018.1540821

Rosenblatt, B. (2014). Museum education and art therapy: Promoting wellness in older adults. *Journal of Museum Education*, *39*(3), 293–301.

Rubin, J. (2010). *Introduction to art therapy: Sources and resources*. New York: Routledge.

Salom, A. (2015). Weaving potential space and acculturation: Art therapy at the museum. *Journal of Applied Arts & Health*, *6*(1), 47–62.

Seligman, M. (2011). *Flourish: A visionary new understanding of happiness and well-being*. New York: Free Press.

Silverman, L. H. (2010). *The social work of museums*. New York: Routledge.

Thaler, L., Drapeau, C., Leclerc, J., Lajeunesse, M., Cottier, D., Kahan, E., Ferenczy, N. & Steiger, H. (2017). An adjunctive, museum-based art therapy experience in the treatment of women with severe eating disorders. *The Arts in Psychotherapy*, *56*, 1–6.

Treadon, C. B., Rosal, M. & Thompson Wylder, V. D. (2006). Opening the doors of art museums for therapeutic processes. *The Arts in Psychotherapy*, *33*(4), 288–301. DOI:10.1016/j.aip.2006.03.003

Wilkinson, R. & Chilton, G. (2018). *Positive art therapy: Theory and practice*. New York: Routledge.

Winnicott, D. (1971). *Playing and reality*. London: Tavistock/Routledge.

4   Museum-based Art Therapy

A Collaborative Effort with Access, Education, and Public Programming

Mitra Reyhani Ghadim

My museum art therapy trajectory was shaped by approaches in art therapy, and by research and theories in museum education, schools, and libraries. Over the years of community work, I increasingly appreciated the important role of inviting institutions such as museums and libraries in community care and wellness. I was inspired by the work of David Carr, who wrote:

> There are many possibilities of experience in an inviting institution: we absorb, hold, assemble, connect, construct; we fabricate; we plan, we expect, we anticipate, we hope; we hypothesize, infer, assume, fantasize; we ask, pause, converse, clarify, return and linger, compare, elaborate, recollect; we remember and evoke; we discover and surrender, we become.
>
> (2006, p. 28)

Museum-based art therapy projects that I was involved in were developed with the idea that community-based services can thrive by transforming museums into *inviting institutions* for all members of various communities. "As we thread the needle of our thoughts, we stitch the fabric of experience" (Carr, 2006, p. 28), and museums can offer platforms for new experience for visitors, as well as fields of experimentation for art therapy, access, and education fields.

The Museum: An Inviting Institution

My practice as a museum art therapist began a decade ago with a graduate art therapy program internship placement at the Queens Museum of Art (now Queens Museum) in New York. At the time – in 2011 – the site already had an art therapy program (called Art*Access*) and autism initiatives, with two full-time art therapists and one part-time one. This established art therapy program was receiving ongoing support and encouragement from the museum's executive director of the time, Tom Finkelpearl, who had a unique vision of *openness* for the museum. As I understand it, the concept of openness was not only about the idea of cooperative thinking, planning, and implementing with the community, but it also involved something empowering and visionary for us as museum workers: a democratic openness to museum staff's ideas and visions

DOI: 10.4324/9781003014386-4

around museums and their role in social justice and social practice, education, access, and community service. This view made itself visible in the way we, as museum professionals, were granted autonomy for forming and implementing our ideas to address social issues by planning and structuring programs in accordance with our departmental specialties. These specialties were school programs, adult and teen programs, art therapy (all ages), public programs, community organizing, and curatorship. The one-word concept of openness invited individual ideas of staff and the community to envision what a museum can be and how we can have a proactive role in the well-being of communities, as well as in the promotion of social justice.

Within this museum landscape, art therapists were considered to have an essential role in connecting with and serving diverse neighboring communities and organizations in Queens, New York, as well as other boroughs and Long Island. Through these encounters and the collective meaning-making by art therapists and clients, community-based art therapy initiatives were generated together, with, and for the community (Dejkameh & Sabbaghi, 2019).

In this chapter, I share information based on my experience gained as a full-time art therapist involved in numerous art therapy projects and initiatives, hoping to disseminate useful knowledge for art therapists interested in working in or collaborating with museums. In the last 4 years of my time as the manager, during which the program grew, I generally worked simultaneously on multiple projects, together with one or more full-time art therapists, two or more part-time art therapists/coordinators, and an average of 14 art therapists and/or educators and teaching artists who were contractually on the program roster.

We created programs for diverse populations including children, adolescents, adults, older adults, and families. These museum-based art therapy projects were implemented in collaboration with mental health agencies, school districts, community programs, residential treatment programs, hospitals, correctional facilities, and wellness centers. The autism initiative of the art therapy program provided sessions for children with autism and their siblings, parents, or guardians. Other examples from autism initiatives were multiyear museum internship programs and a bimonthly Open Art Studio for young adults with autism.

All on-site sessions were facilitated at the museum's Studio B, a large studio equipped with sinks and storage. The studio was dedicated to the art therapy program, which helped us maintain its safety and accessibility for all participating populations. We facilitated our off-site sessions in community-based settings and offered remote virtual programs to homebound seniors and nursing homes (2016–2018).

Museum Art Therapy, an Interdisciplinary Enterprise

The critical work of Silverman created a shift in the way museums are viewed by moving away from conceiving museums as spaces where educators work on effective transmission of ideas, to spaces where visitors create meanings (1995). Access and education departments have increasingly explored opportunities to make individual meanings and worldviews of visitors and program participants more visible in the larger social discourse. As art therapy and museum education are both rooted in goals of promoting dialogue when looking at art objects (Grandison, 2020), museums and cultural institutions are ideal territories for initiating discussions for individual or collaborative meaning construction through art looking and artmaking.

Aside from self-directed open studio format programs at the Queens Museum, art therapists created museum art therapy directives for school partnership sessions and other organizations. These were designed in ways that aimed for the inclusion of individuals of different abilities, individuals with varying cultural, socioeconomic backgrounds, and individuals in special situations. This unique practice often involved collaboration with other museum professionals. It was also informed by its surrounding communities and its visitors' needs or interests. At the time, the education department of the Queens Museum was the largest department of the museum (until leadership changes in 2019), consisting of the following four specialized programs, each led by one full-time manager and one or more full- or part-time coordinators:

1.   School programs (SPs)
2.   Art therapy programs: Art*Access* and autism initiatives (AA)
3.   Family, after-school, teens, and out-of-school programs (OST)
4.   New New Yorkers programs (programs for adult immigrants; NNY)

These programs had ongoing dialogues and intersected frequently, with staff working together in ways that could benefit different visitors. Collaborative projects involved working with one or more programs from the above-mentioned education team of school, family/after-school/teens team, adult programs – as well as interdepartmentally with public programs and the curatorial team. In the next two sections I give a brief description of case examples for two collaborative projects.

Case Example 1: Communiversity of Inclusive Play

Studies around social inclusion and museums demonstrate links between loss of identity and social exclusion, and that museum-based community development projects can enable participants to create new social identities through shared experiences (Newman & Mclean, 2006). An example of a collaborative project with other museum departments, outside organizations, and community participants was the Communiversity of Inclusive Play, a project involving the participation of 21 families who had children with disabilities. This 18-month project was funded by the National Art Education Association. As its title of *Communiversity* reflects, the project was designed to become a learning experience with the involvement of parents and caregivers, and to have a positive impact on identifying strengths of participating families. All but one family were Spanish-speaking; therefore, simultaneous translations and other printed support were provided throughout the program period.

A public playground in the vicinity of the museum was an outdoor space that was central to this project. This outdoor space, the Playground for All Children in Flushing Meadows Corona Park was the first NYC playground with accessibility for all children, including those with disabilities, designed and opened in 1984. In making the playground central to the art therapy project, we wanted families to have a significant presence in the surrounding community through artmaking projects stationed in the public playground, and for them to become more visible within their sociocultural context through art. This program involved partnership between several museum departments (art therapy, public programs, out-of-school, and after-school programs), the Parks Department, the Queens College Psychology Department, and families who had children with disabilities. Nature inspires people to go beyond routine responses and to connect with the greater biosphere inhabited by other livings things (Whitaker, 2010). The artmaking stations in the public playground used natural elements to spark new ways of connecting with the world.

Twenty-one families who had children with disabilities registered to participate in this project. Families signed a contract and consent form and were offered an honorarium for their participation as well as subway cards for their commuting.

We asked the following leading questions for Communiversity for Inclusive Play:

1. How can a learning community support families who have children with disabilities?
2. How can a public space such as a community playground be activated as a site for a new, inclusive model for arts-based participation and learning?

To find answers to these questions, we structured the program with two components: *Family Institutes* and *Public Playground Programs*. Family Institutes included 12 learning sessions for families with one or more children with disabilities. These training sessions were offered to support families by connecting them with various institutional resources, and to introduce community-based art therapy and other inclusive and accessible activities for children with disabilities. Public programs took place once a month at the Playground for All Children. Coordinated with the NYC Parks Department, these Sunday programs were structured to offer six art workshops stationed throughout various areas of the playground on each date. Activity stations were collaboratively planned and prepared for in the museum with families and facilitated by art therapists and teaching artists together with parents. Participating families' children, as well as other children visiting the playground, were invited to create art in various stations.

Communiversity was a rich collaboration between the museum's innovations: long-term engagement with social practice artists, full-time art therapists creatively working with children with disabilities, and a full-time community organizer who partners with artists to support local organizing movements, including efforts around public spaces. Sunday events in the Playground for All Children took place over two summers and were an opportunity for an innovative art-based partnership with the Parks Department using outdoor spaces. The program offered informative workshops for parents, providing them with various types of information that could be useful in finding and navigating resources in the community, including accessing therapy and enrichment program resources for their child from various organizations. Another part of the sessions aimed to advance creative ideas for the community playground's transformation into a more inclusive and family-friendly space through planning structured art workshops based on parent suggestions. While parent institutes and planning workshops were in session in one studio, other art therapists and interns worked with their children in the art studio that was adjacent to the space where parents participated in training and planning sessions.

Along with training for parents at the museum and collaborative dialogues with them about creative activities they would like to see their children participate in, they were gradually gaining confidence as they were practicing and preparing for co-leading and later leading Sunday stations in the Playground for all Children. With the guidance of art therapists, educators, community organizers, and two parent leaders, they all became involved in creating art and facilitating art workshops, as well as dance/movement and nature exploration programs in the playground every month throughout these two consecutive summers. Examples of parents' interesting directive ideas included dance and movement. Parents also created a soil and planting directive where children would write wishes on papers that were placed with seeds. This directive was a metaphor for the growth and actualization of a wish or goal. On each date in the playground program, five or six activity stations would be set in the playground, all designed to be accessible, flexible, and adaptive to all 21 families' children, ages 7–21, with varying physical or developmental disabilities. Projects were designed to be engaging, empowering, and therapeutic. These stations were open for about 3.5 hours on the Sundays when programs were offered. Communiversity of Inclusive Play was anchored by an in-depth art therapy experience geared toward the family members of young people with disabilities living in the vicinity of the Playground for All Children to have a more visible presence in their public playground and offering them opportunities to practice leadership roles through art and mutual support. Over several months, families became increasingly involved in decision-making and taking initiatives as co-leaders and leaders.

Another outcome of Communiversity was a *Fotonovela* project, created based on a story written by parents to express the challenges of stigmatization they face in their daily lives. The plot of the story was acted, photographed by participating children and parents, and printed by museum staff. *Fotonovela* contributed to the empowerment of families by allowing them to share common issues as a supportive group.

In summary, Communiversity had the significant impact of creating a supportive community by bringing together 21 Spanish-speaking families who had children with disabilities and involving them in a yearlong collaboration leading to networking, support, and increased knowledge. It spoke to the larger goal and impact of art therapy in social practice and empowerment. Many families remained connected by communicating and planning through social media networking beyond the project period. They continued to collaborate through networking, supporting each other to advance the goal of inclusivity through ongoing community outreach through other initiatives and by organizing projects.

Case Example 2: Parent Ambassadors in Visitor Experience

The Parent Ambassadors in Visitor Experience (PAVE) project was designed to help local families who have younger children, with and without disabilities alike, engage in self-directed, experiential learning in the museum galleries, and to enable the visitor-facing staff to better understand the needs of the diverse families visiting the museum galleries.

For this project, we reached out to a local partner elementary school's PTA to coordinate and share information about the initiative with parents and caregivers. Small groups of families participated in art programs with art therapists and the museum's visitor experience agents. In this project, we collaborated interdepartmentally with our frontline staff visitor experience department as well as the family program within the education department.

During PAVE, families experimented with different ways art can support learning and development in the museum by making museum galleries more inviting for families who have young children, with or without disabilities. With the coordinators of the program, Rachel Shipps and Jennifer Candiano, we asked the question: "How can we support parents to be self-directed in creating memorable learning experiences with their families in the museum galleries?" To answer this question, we looked at various tools and techniques we already used as museum art therapists and we considered how those could be utilized in this project.

The project consisted of four consecutive 3-month cycles. Each cycle's participants consisted of six families who had children ages 4–12. A total of 24 families participated throughout the four cycles. Each cycle's structure included:

1. An introductory session
2. Parent leadership workshops in which museum staff professionals and outside experts shared creative methods with parents for engaging their children in the galleries

3. Artmaking and art-looking workshops for parents and children
4. The planning and execution of a culminating family day at the museum

PAVE made museum galleries more engaging spaces for families in inspiring art experiences, regardless of their linguistic abilities and art historical knowledge. After the completion of the four cycles, we produced a printed guide, *Paving New Ways of Exploration in Cultural Institutions* (Dejkameh, Candiano, & Shipps, 2018), as a tool for internal training of visitor experience agents and a resource for families as well as other cultural institutions offering best practices for engaging families with children ages 4–12. Collaborating project partners that were instrumental in planning and in spreading the word about the project throughout their expansive networks were:

1. Cool Culture, an organization that ensures New York City's most diverse families with preschool-aged children have access to arts and culture to increase literacy and learning in early childhood.
2. The Engaging Educator, an organization that provides workshops that improve presentation skills, storytelling abilities, and communication skills through improv-based techniques.
3. Yadira De La Riva, an artist, activist, and performer, who led the professional development on improvised, performative techniques and games in the Spanish language.

Although originally conceived of as a family programs initiative, it was discovered that the skill set of the art therapy program was better suited to promote parent-led learning in the galleries for families with young children, and the art therapy program team gained more leadership of PAVE. This project increased family engagement in the museum galleries by engaging 39 families, 43 parents, and 57 children, which was more than we had anticipated.

Through art therapy methods, we worked with parents on practicing how to make personal connections to art for meaning-making and to use strategies to allow their children to make similar connections. We used accessibility and educational methods such as universal design for learning (UDL) and positive behavior support (PBS) to emphasize activity and experimentation through engagement. By emphasizing that personal responses and reactions of participants were central to arts engagement (as opposed to art historical knowledge), we successfully demonstrated to local parents that cultural institutions can be incredible resources for engaging their children in enriching, fun activities. Improv-based professional development sessions were integrated with art therapy methods and were particularly useful in demonstrating nonverbal and alternative methods that increase the ability of the mind to learn in the classroom and beyond (Flanagan, 2015) and allow deeper engagement in inclusive arts-based activities for families visiting museums with young children.

Our Interdisciplinary Approach

Positive Behavior
Support (PBS)

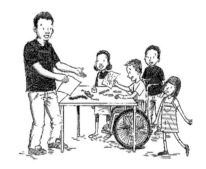

Art Therapy

Universal Design for
Learning (UDL)

Applied Behavior Analysis (ABA)

Museum Education Strategies
(Inquiry-Based; Visual Thinking VTS)

Figure 4.1 Interdisciplinary approach in museum art therapy

Illustration by Paul Hoppe

I agree with Kapitan who wrote that art therapists have limitless potential for creating new forms in the worlds that are life-enhancing, but that they may hold a vision of their practice that is driven by a longing to align with established categories of mental health care as well as those recognized by the art world (2003). We implemented other museum art therapy initiatives that went beyond the typical museum art therapy programming to address accessibility, equity, and social justice. Some of these programs were multi-year internship programs for young adults with disabilities and virtual exhibitions, sessions for individuals who were homebound. The following two sections offer readers information about such projects.

Internship Opportunities for Young Adults with ASD

Adults with ASD who attended public schools and grew up with their families are members of a community and need to develop independence within the community (Gonzalez-Dolginko, 2020). After several years of working in partnership with middle and high school students with autism, we became increasingly interested in creating opportunities for young adults with disabilities so they can learn to cope and integrate in work settings. A major goal for their treatment is to offer support and enhance coping skills as they move toward independence in post-school life (Gonzalez-Dolginko, 2020), and we thought working as interns in the museum would be a safe way for high school-age individuals with ASD to experiment with this important treatment goal. We applied for funding and established contracts that would allow museum art therapists to work on creating programs to benefit young adults with disabilities as they transition to post-school life, and we initiated internship programs that we were able to sustain for several years. The overall goals for museum internships were:

- Creating community-based art experiences for high school students with disabilities and with varying skills to support their transition to post-school life
- Forming an internship program model through which individuals with diverse physical, developmental, and learning abilities make contributions to art and knowledge, making the museum a space where art and social justice intersect

Specific objectives were:

- Providing interns with disabilities with the opportunity to experience a sense of mastery and accomplishment in the museum community
- Creating and implementing an arts-based curriculum so interns can identify and use their specific skills and interests in a work-like setting and learn about art careers in cultural institutions
- Providing opportunities for interns to practice, with the support of art therapy techniques, interpersonal skills they can employ in their post-school life

We implemented the first PrintShop Internship program (2015) through a VSA Rosemary Kennedy Internship contract. During an academic year, museum art therapists worked with interns with autism on creating monoprints using foam plates or linoleum for various sellable products such as T-shirts, canvas bags, art paper, and other materials. Interns were periodically provided with opportunities where they sold their artistic products in a community market. The museum's annual holiday market provided another platform for them to practice interacting and selling their work. A year later, through the Skill-Based Internship program, we provided intensive internship experience for high school students with ASD. This project was multifaceted, and one of its final outcomes was a video documentary made by interns with ASD about their yearlong internship experience. Interns were trained in various arts-based vocational activities such as curating an art exhibit for their high school's annual art exhibition in the museum's partnership gallery, creating invitation cards for the exhibit, and creating résumé and artist statements in pamphlets that they would distribute during these events at their schools. These activities addressed many skills, some relating to socialization, others to learning new knowledge through art and arts-based projects such as curating art which required measuring and gathering other information about artworks.

To develop exceptional internship experiences for individuals with ASD, we started with gradual steps by first using computer-based career tests to learn about each intern's area of interest. We also sent questionnaires to families to learn about their child's out-of-school interests and activities so we can use their input. Each artist received an art journal for daily entry of their thoughts, feelings, and what may have captured their interest in the galleries. We then largely focused on practicing interviewing skills through role-play. Another significant part of their curriculum was focused on photography, filming, word processing, and graphic art. These techniques were practiced through carefully structured sessions using many visual prompts. Each internship session was facilitated by an art therapist and a teaching artist who would collaboratively design each structured session. We used a visual vocabulary for each session, and students who did not speak used an iPad for communication, with the Proloquo2Go application, a user-friendly platform where art therapists were able to add additional themes/images for each session. As part of their sessions, some of the activities interns with ASD engaged in included:

1. Practicing interviewing one another, then meeting, interviewing, and filming various departments' staff
2. Taking on responsibilities during their school's culminating event, which 15 classes with students with disabilities attended. Each intern was responsible for a station during the 2-hour event: photo booth, prop handler, snack table, program distribution, and guiding classes to the theater and inviting them to watch the documentary they had made about their internship

After many years of contracted, funded internship initiatives, we had developed a clear and generalizable structure that we then applied to new incoming interns with disabilities from Queens College Special Inclusion Program.

Tele-art Therapy with Individuals who Are Homebound

Between 2016 and 2018, the art therapy program of the museum offered *tele-art therapy* sessions for individuals who were homebound. The project allowed participants to explore programs that were safe and stimulating and offered opportunities for expression and self-actualization. The project was implemented in partnership with the Queens Library branch which offered mail-a-book and other programs for older adults. Library partnerships were part of the art therapy program's ongoing engagement with formal and informal learning experiences in museums and libraries.

We drew inspiration from museum exhibits to provide teleconferences and Zoom video conferences to older adults who were homebound through a partnership with Queens Library funded by the Institute of Museum and Library Services (IMLS). Every 2 weeks, participants who registered through the library received large-print booklets on museum exhibit images and art kits that they later processed during Zoom and teleconferences with museum educators and art therapists. Sessions were facilitated in English and Mandarin for populations who spoke each language. Since the onset of the COVID-19 pandemic, looking at many museum programs as well as other art therapy programs largely relying on Zoom and other digital platforms, we can see how the 2016–18 Zoom-based, museum tele-art therapy programs we implemented were innovative and visionary. Some Zoom-based virtual sessions were facilitated in front of select artworks in the galleries and individuals from library branches, as well as nursing homes, through which participants could join for real-time Zoom discussions.

General Museum Art Therapy Approaches

As some of our programs were facilitated in the dedicated Studio B of the museum and some off-site in various community locations, the concept of the flexible studio model helped us think about how spaces can become adaptable and responsive, with potential to be activated by participants. Some of the essential strategies we used for designing therapeutic and educational programs and environments included *universal design for learning*, *positive behavior support*, and *project-based learning*, each briefly described below.

Universal Design for Learning

We used UDL as a model premised on the idea that all people should be able to use all products and spaces. Its objectives align with art therapy strategies, including sessions that address the needs of individuals with varying learning styles by using the following three principles:

1.   Multiple and flexible means of representation
2.   Multiple and flexible ways of expression
3.   Multiple and flexible ways of engagement

As museum art therapists, we considered participants with various disabilities, developmental levels, and learning styles when developing directives, using multiple flexible ways of representation and engagement (Figure 4.2). We used these principles to guide us for studio layout, accessibility of materials, and structuring the sessions.

In designing sessions with UDL principles in mind, we included techniques to go beyond what might typically be used with a specific population. For example, when working with individuals who are blind or have low vision, in addition to the common use of clay or other 3D material for sculpture or textured paint for painting, we took advantage of having a print press machine in the studio and created a series of sessions using the embossing techniques (Figure 4.3).

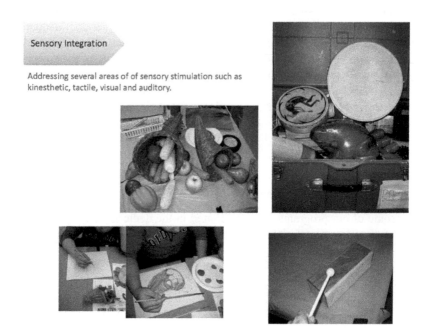

Sensory Integration

Addressing several areas of of sensory stimulation such as kinesthetic, tactile, visual and auditory.

Figure 4.2 Multiple flexible ways of representation

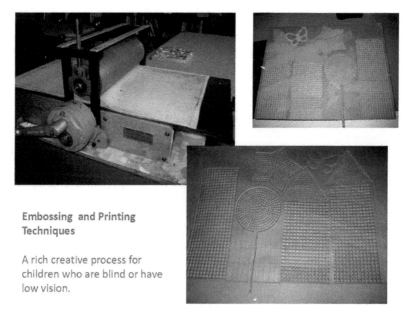

Embossing and Printing Techniques

A rich creative process for children who are blind or have low vision.

Figure 4.3 Embossing techniques

Positive Behavior Support

Based on values and empirical research, PBS provides a process to understand and address challenging behavior in individuals, including children. It helps create understanding of why an individual engages in behavior and suggests strategies to work with individuals who may display difficult behavior. PBS offers a holistic, proactive approach that aligns with art therapy by considering all factors that have an impact on the individual's behavior.

Project-based Learning (PBL)

Project-based learning (PBL) is a method in which individuals develop critical-thinking, problem-solving, collaboration, and self-management skills by investigating and responding to a complex, engaging question, problem, or challenge. Project-based learning allows for learning by doing (Dewey, 1997), and learners and facilitators engage in collaborative activities to find solutions to questions of interest that mirror skills and competencies that experts use in solving problems (Krajcik & Shin, 2014). The method gives value to the project using real-world context and by speaking to the individual's personal concerns, interests, and issues, and all of these approaches align with art therapy techniques that emphasize individual questions and foster problem-solving skills and subjective meaning-making during therapeutic encounters.

Adaptive Tools
ABA Method

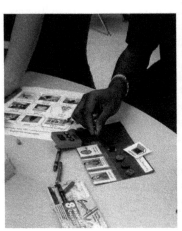
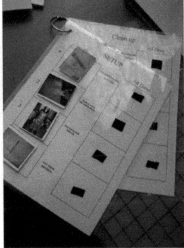

Figure 4.4 Visual vocabulary and setup/cleanup sheets

In creating open, flexible, safe spaces inside the museum galleries, we used the same basic ideas that we had developed in the studio to help us access all learners at different age or developmental levels. The visual vocabulary tool was developed in 2011 by the program's art therapists and refined since then to support sessions with children pre-K–12 with autism, students who are nonverbal, and/or children and adults as diverse learners. Creating a visual vocabulary sheet for each session offers a flexible way of representation for sessions. The visual vocabulary can contain both concrete (museum, educator, paint, brush) and abstract (collage, friendship, disassemble) ideas. This tool and other visual tools were used when working with schools where the ABA-based behavioral method is used to make the sessions easily accessible for students with autism (Figure 4.4).

Conclusion and Final Notes

Museum-based art therapy is not simply an isolated or clinically oriented practice that is situated within a cultural institution. It is, rather, a cumulative formation of community-based practice informed by the intersection of several disciplines. The knowledge gathered for the implementation of museum art therapy is derived from a hybrid of wellness, education, access, and public programs. Relational reflexivity and pedagogical approaches form conceptual frameworks for the development and growth of museum art therapy programs for various populations. Based on our experience of adapting a studio space in various types of community-based settings, we also created engaging spaces in the galleries to transform the entire museum into a space for sharing, relaxing, gathering, and making.

These innovative projects continued until 2019, when change in the education department leadership as well as the executive leadership led to a sudden decrease in all programs of the education department as well as public programs, leading to staff resignations. The new approach proved to be different than the previous one that invited museum workers to contribute their visions. This unfortunate situation was even more exacerbated by the COVID-19 pandemic, when many more frontline and educator staff were laid off.

With the occurrence of the pandemic, as art therapy practitioners we have been witnessing art therapy in some platforms decreasing, but opportunities for new programs and platforms have been given to us. A nomadic adaptation requires strategies that will recreate the therapeutic space by learning from each territory and adapting to it to engage participants in new and evolving physical and virtual spaces. Over time, we can continue to create and refine new models for in-person as well as virtual experiences that are flexible, safe, and accessible for many populations.

References

Carr, D. (2006). *A place not a place: Reflection and possibility in museums and libraries*. Lanham, MD: Alta Mira Press.

Dejkameh, M., Candiano, J. & Shipps, R. (2018). *Paving new ways of exploration in cultural institutions: A gallery guide for inclusive arts-based engagement in cultural institutions*. Queens Museum

Dejkameh, M. & Sabbaghi, V. (2019). From please touch to Art*Access*, a rhizomatic growth. In A. Wexler & V. Sabbaghi (Eds.), *Bridging communities through socially engaged art* (57–66). New York, NY: Routledge.

Dewey, J. (1997). Experience and education. New York: Touchstone.

Flanagan, L. (2015). How improv can open up the mind to learning in the classroom and beyond. www.kqed.org/mindshift/39108/how-improv-can-open-up-the-mind-to-learning-in-the-classroom-and-beyond

Gonzalez-Dolginko, B. (2020). *Art therapy with adults with autism spectrum disorder*. Jessica Kingsley.

Grandison, S. (2020). Expanding the frame, developing, and sustaining a long term NHS art museum partnership within a workforce development strategy for enhanced quality of care. In A. Coles & H. Jury (Eds.), *Art therapy in museums and galleries* (181–201). Jessica Kingsley.

Murphy P. A. (2014). Let's Move! How Body Movements Drive Learning Through Technology.

Kapitan, L. (2003). *Re-enchanting art therapy: Transformational practices for restoring creative vitality*. Springfield, IL: Charles C. Thomas.

Krajcik, J. S. & Shin, N. (2014). Project-based learning. In K. Sawyer (Ed.), *The Cambridge handbook of learning sciences* (275–297). Cambridge University Press.

Newman A. & McLean, F. (2006). The impact of museums upon identity. *International Journal of Heritage Studies*, *12*(1), 49–68.

Silverman, L. (1995). Visitor meaning making for a new age. *Curator*, *38*(3), 161–170.

Whitaker, P. (2010). Groundswell: The nature and landscape of art therapy. In C. H. Monn (Ed.), *Materials and media in art therapy: Critical understandings of diverse artistic vocabularies* (119–136). Routledge.

5 A Binational Participatory Project with Families Affected by Autism in the Museum Art Therapy Context

Michelle López Torres and Mitra Reyhani Ghadim

Introduction

Cultural institutions can function as supportive mediators for the participation and construction of knowledge with families affected by autism through programs that engage them in the arts. This view is in alignment with Freire who wrote, "To teach is not to transfer knowledge but to create the possibilities for the production or construction of knowledge" (Freire, 1998, p. 30). As contemporary art increasingly gravitates to issues related to social justice, global, and environmental concerns, the role of the art therapist working in a cultural institution is increasingly informed by the principles of social action, socially engaged art, participatory research, and ethnography. The role of the art therapist in initiating and carrying out programs in the education department of a museum may be compared to transactions that take place in a public library in New York. In a library, the service offered is nonjudgmental, non-privileged, and egalitarian (Carr, 2011). In a cultural institution, similarly, service is ideally designed to respond to a community's needs. The public library's goal is to address the community's character and needs and to anticipate its changes (Carr, 2014). A cultural institution with a mission that involves a vision for *openness* to diverse ideas of communities will have similar objectives.

One interesting museum art therapy program was the Art*Access* program of Queens Museum. The program began in1983 as Please Touch, originally a special education pilot program designed for children who were blind or had low vision (Reyhani Dejkameh & Shipps, 2019; Peacock, 2012). Since 1983, for almost four decades (1983–2019), Art*Access* expanded significantly to provide services for individuals with physical, visual, speech, hearing, and learning disabilities, as well as those with developmental and emotional diversities (Peacock, 2012). The program also served individuals in special situations (e.g., extended hospitalization, second-hand trauma, and homelessness), and program participants were able to access the museum regardless of an inability to travel, whether they were housed in rehabilitation hospitals or other medically restricted settings; had conditions that required continuous special

DOI: 10.4324/9781003014386-5

care; were in the foster care system; or were in prison or detention (Peacock, 2012). Under the leadership of several art therapists, the Art*Access* program grew, especially in the decade from 2011 until July of 2019. Since then, the program's scope of service has decreased significantly, and its direction has at this time become uncertain owing to changes in the leadership of both the executive and education departments.

This chapter describes one of the many projects designed and implemented by museum art therapists in support of families. Focused on autism, this multiyear family art therapy program was designed and implemented from 2013 to 2015, at the height of the growth of the Art*Access* museum art therapy program. The project described in this chapter was funded by the American Alliance of Museums (AAM) and the State Department for Educational and Cultural Affairs with the collaborative efforts and leadership of six families in Spain and six families in the United States.

Background of the US–Spain Participatory Autism Initiative

Because of pleas from parent advocates, the Royal Spanish Academy (the official royal Spanish institution that ensures the stability of the Spanish language) changed the definition of "autism" in the Spanish language dictionary in 2011. As relayed in one Spanish blog, *Think Spain*, until that time "autism" had been defined as "a condition where those affected were 'incapable' of 'showing affection' or 'giving and feeling love" (*Think Spain*, 2012). This made it terribly upsetting for parents in Spain with a child diagnosed with autism; they believed their own child would never love them.

Spain was then not only experiencing the transformation of what the word autism means, but also how the image of autism was portrayed. Along with the change in definition, the perception of what autism was and how it related to people on a day-to-day basis was also changing. The idea of communicating with their children started appearing to be less impossible to parents in Spain, and the realization that children with autism could show emotions was becoming more prevalent.

Similarly, in 2012, the American Psychiatric Association changed the meaning of autism in the fifth edition of the *Diagnostic and Statistical Manual of Mental Disorders* (DSM-5) to a new definition that changed its diagnostic characteristic in the American medical field. The redefining of autism in the DSM-5 has been leading to changes in treatment protocols and services, leaving parents unsure of what this will mean for the institutionalized services targeted to their child with autism. With the definition of autism in flux, diagnosing a child with autism not only became complex, but seeking support, guidance, and services from cultural institutions once a diagnosis has been made proved just as difficult. Because parents and caregivers should select appropriate programming, it can be hard to decide which methods and activities will work best for their child, as both the diagnosis and the services offered keep changing. The role of the parent as advocate when dealing with a diagnosis as complex as autism has proven necessary time and again; parents are experts in knowing their children's unique personalities.

In New York, with special education reforms (2012–13) returning services back to the family's community, the future of treatments for autism and other types of disability relies greatly on parents. The special education reform of New York intended to provide more students with disabilities access to their zoned schools and other schools of choice. Because of this, most NYC public schools were then expected to meet the needs of their students with individualized education plans (IEPs). Parents had to choose between integration of their children in local schools that may have less specialized equipment and professional services for unique needs, or an NYC District 75 school exclusively for children with multiple and severe disabilities, which offered more accessible technology as well as specialized staff. Although these changes and reforms made for an important civil rights case for people with disabilities, parents often find it daunting to navigate the maze of treatment and educational services. Even with all the right resources, parents have to become better at identifying appropriate education plans for their children. First, however, the resources that help to identify the array of treatment and education plans must be made more accessible to all. All of these changes were discussed in an ongoing manner between us as museum art therapists, parents who had their child participate in our family or our school partnership programs, as well as our partner District 75 schools, teachers, and administrators. Years of exchange and interactions with these communities and organizations planted the seeds for thinking about how the museum can be used as a tool to support families.

The Role of the Museum Art Therapist in emPower Parents Project

Human beings develop in part by responding to contributions from others, and we provide others with materials they can respond to (Eisner, 2012). An art therapist's practice can involve initiating opportunities for parents to become involved in research, becoming deeply engaged in a dynamic process of doing and learning, and contributing their knowledge of self and their child's process with an awareness of their own learning and becoming, or what Freire termed as the unfinished-ness of self and the openness to the new (1998). Permanent openness to engaging in participatory projects and exchange with clients is the correct attitude for one who does not consider her/himself to be the only possessor of truth or the passive object of ideology or gossip (Freire, 1998). In the work of apprenticeship that the art therapist undertakes, this openness can be applied in dealing with all members of a community. With this openness, the art therapist can be freed from the influence of established cultural and theoretical dominance (Reyhani Ghadim, 2020) and creatively use various settings for innovative art therapy programs. The art therapist's role in a community-based setting is critical in detecting and making contributions to new transformations in established cultural themes that may inhibit creative thinking in populations considered marginal or outsiders by a system. Kapitan, Litell, and Torres (2011) defined art as an act of critical consciousness, evoking new ways of thinking and learning that things can change (Kapitan et al., 2011). Art can function as a tool to achieve the inclusion of creative voices and unique worlds of all members of society.

The emPower Parents museum art therapy project was initiated at a time when both Spain and the United States were facing similar concerns about the development of educational and enrichment programming for autism, as well as changes in the way autism is seen and approached. ABA-based behavioral services were not covered by health or education services in Spain (Keenan et al., 2015). There had been a few documented exceptions where a court had mandated that a particular individual should receive intensive behavioral intervention. All services for autism were almost always paid for privately by families (Keenan et al., 2015). In the United States, most families cannot afford to hire their own specialists to help their children, and they look to public school special education programs for these services (McLaughlin, 2017). Both countries had experienced a change in the definition of autism and, along with that, changes in the amenities offered to people diagnosed and their families. With these changes, participating parents in Spain and the United States – more specifically, in Madrid and Queens – had shown the desire and will to advocate for their children so they could have greater participation in social and creative programs.

As art therapists who aim to determine the next useful strategy for our museum-based practice, we wanted to have a general openness to explore multiple realities and perspectives. This would allow for a democratic relationship with community members. The nature of our work allowed us to be in a position to offer a more humane, less commodity-oriented, and more relationship-based view of art (Moon, 2003). The art therapist's role in engaging with communities became a moving, nomadic role (Reyhani Ghadim, 2020), following points that determined the pathways. What determined our pathway to build a closer exchange through a binational project with parents affected by autism was the idea that such an exchange can inform our practice with and for the population affected by autism spectrum disorders.

Asking themself systematic key questions can engage a community-based art therapist in a process of self-reflection when working in a setting that does not offer policies and procedures for establishing therapeutic goals (Elmendorf, 2010). The systematic questions asked throughout this project were informed by years of experience of previous programming that was designed for families affected by autism who participated in the Museum Explorers Club program, as well as results obtained from collaborative action research on various other art therapy programs in the museum throughout the years. The language the museum art therapist uses to ask systematic questions will not necessarily sound like the language of "therapy" or "treatment" common to a mental health setting or other clinical settings, but will rather be focused on the process of articulating answers to key questions, allowing community-based art therapists to facilitate art-making experiences while ensuring basic ethical principles (Elmendorf, 2010). The questions we asked were generally around the positive effects of making the museum programs universally accessible and encouraging the participation of the whole family in rich art sessions in the museum context to create an inclusive and integrated interactive environment. The above-mentioned Museum Explorers Club was a family program facilitated on weekends for several years by museum art therapists. Families who had children with autism participated each Saturday. Siblings, parents, and grandparents were invited to participate and to be part of the museum art therapy sessions. This approach had generated especially inclusive dynamics, and children socially interacted with each other's siblings and families through fun, engaging, and educational weekly sessions with both gallery and studio components.

Over years of programming, we learned from families that parents' access to both information on and resources for the variety of treatment and education plans for their children with autism is crucial. With a more positive prognosis, images of families engaging in activities together and building memories while taking intervention into their own creative hands were becoming more common. As noted before, the transformation that the meaning of the word "autism" was undergoing had been a long process that required education and the support of cultural institutions. Involving families in this creative process could help them develop their own ways of communication to express their needs, and they could in turn experience great success in reaching and empowering their diverse community members through art. Therefore, by initiating the emPower Parents participatory project, as art therapists we hoped to initiate dialogues and communication that would result in greater understanding of the mutual strengths and needs of parents in the U.S. and Spain. We also hoped it would lead participants toward empowerment, encouraging them to become leaders and create desired change in their communities.

Method

With awards from the State Department and the American Alliance of Museums, the emPower Parents participatory project allowed art therapists to collaborate with families affected by autism in Queens, New York, and Madrid, Spain, along with other communities and organizations in both countries. The emPower Parents binational museum art therapy project was conducted within a participatory action research (PAR) framework. PAR is a process of inquiry conducted by all participants involved in a project who work together to investigate common questions or problems and can result in new knowledge for the purpose of making change, with the facilitator supporting group cohesion and collective inquiry (Kapitan, 2010). The project consisted of many elements, holding an international value of collaboration and exchange.

As a construct, the project was initiated through ongoing open discussions and collaborative decision-making. This structure called for new ideas and questions to emerge from the participants throughout the year. With participatory orientation, the researcher renounces the role of expert in favor of the shared knowledge and expertise of the group as a whole (Kapitan, 2010). Sharing of knowledge becomes an ongoing mutual enterprise throughout the collaboration. Ideas about collaborating with Spain-based families who have children with autism originated and grew and were gradually shaped through discussions with families who had previously participated in our family programs.

This method followed a cyclical mode of inquiry that is based on applying new knowledge obtained from taking action to practice. It involved a series of "action, reflection, action" steps that allowed for examining a problem or situation that needed improvement, developing a hypothesis and testing it, observing and examining the outcomes critically, then reformulating the hypothesis, taking further action, and subsequently reflecting on its effectiveness to produce change (Kapitan, 2010, p. 98). We had an interest in participatory action because we wanted to test out our actions and implement change by involving families affected by autism in the U.S. and Spain. The challenges were to be redefined by parents and cultural organizations in Spain, allowing for a larger scope and global sense and perspectives. In this way, further dialogues could be created even after the project time line, and support could potentially continue through digital platforms in the future, leading to multiplication and strengthening of community change agents through a form of civic engagement.

Co-participants: Facilitators and Community Participants

The Queens Museum in Queens, New York, Museo ICO, and the cultural organization hablarenarte of Madrid, Spain, collaborated on this 1-year project with the goal to use the initiative Art*Access*, this time in both the U.S. and Spain, to provide an arena that promotes and strengthens advocacy.

Although Museo ICO did not have a formalized program for people with disabilities, in 2011 the Museo furthered its collaboration with the cultural organization hablarenarte to develop programming within the museum space for participants with diverse abilities, including those with autism. hablarenarte was an independent platform for projects and worked to support the creation, publicizing, dissemination, and promotion of contemporary culture (hablarenarte, 2012). This collaboration resulted in the implementation of an education department pilot that invited groups with special needs to each exhibition of Museo ICO for adaptive workshops and tours. Given both museums' track records in engaging participants with disabilities and their demonstrated strength in collaborating with other programs, organizations, and community members, the decision for the two museums to collaborate was a natural progression. This was especially the case given the number of Spanish-speaking families participating in and developing previous programming with Art*Access*, making the language difference less of a barrier.

We expected each party to gain and benefit from this proposed collaboration. In Spain, parents were often on the outside of cultural institutions, working to make changes within the institutions so that they would be more inclusive. For this reason, families with children with autism in Spain, evidenced by the families working with hablarenarte, had demonstrated a very strong parent voice because of a lack of systematic inclusive art programming. They had also demonstrated skills in researching and developing their own tools without institutional help. Parents with children with autism working with the Queens Museum stood to gain an increased sense of civic engagement and parent advocacy. Our hope was that the more empowered parent participants would feel, the more they would take on leadership roles to make institutionalized change for their children, in addition to actively working with the network of community programs as learning partners and consultants.

Structure of the emPower Parents Project within a PAR Methodology

The emPower Parents initiative involved the participation of a group of parents at both the Queens Museum in New York and Museo ICO in Madrid, offering the opportunity to identify and exchange the skills required to request stronger programming and develop education plans for their children with autism.

The structure of this collaborative project comprised two interwoven parts: emPower Parents training and emPower Parents family workshops. Through the training component, parents used the museum as a place to bring awareness to issues around services, programming, and perspectives relating to autism faced by families, and as a place to collaborate with museum art therapists for creative problem-solving. In the family workshop component, art therapists shared structures of their museum art therapy programs, which were informed by interdisciplinary work between the fields of art, art therapy, museum education, and applied behavior analysis techniques. These workshops took place on Skype, simultaneously engaging participants in both the U.S. and Spain.

The project included two initial 6-day retreats during its early weeks, one retreat for each team in the other team's country, and two final 3-day retreats at the end of the 1-year project, with select members traveling to the other team members' country. There were six families participating from the U.S. and six families from Spain. The yearlong project was launched with the previously mentioned 6-day retreat, where three staff participants from the Queens Museum and three families from the U.S. traveled to Madrid, Spain. During this time, participants were able to meet and learn about education and access-based programming for the community in cultural institutions, methods for working with children with autism in Madrid, as well as learning about the meaning and function of the concept of "community" in both countries.

To gain a better understanding of universal feelings about "family," during the first meeting, museum art therapists proposed an art therapy directive with the theme "Family" (Figure 5.1). The project facilitated exchanges and expedited the growth of new friendships among the teams of families and professionals from the U.S. and Spain. This process was essential to create a new binational community of practice, which would have been a challenge without the use of art considering our short period of stay in Madrid and existing language barriers. With the art therapy directive, each family expressed their thoughts and feelings by creating an image of their family using an art medium of their choice. This directive helped us learn about each family's values, as well as supporting the initial group formation efforts of the teams of staff in the U.S. and in Spain.

The first intensive 3-day retreat at Museo ICO supported the shaping of our mutual premise, which was extending each party's knowledge, experience, and available resources to the other and examining how strengthening leadership and advocacy in families and professionals can lead to new strategies in creating art programming that will support families affected by autism. The first day of the 3-day retreat was dedicated to learning about each other at a personal and professional level and sharing insights; the focus of the second day was on learning about our respective professional and community practices for individuals with diverse abilities; and on the third day we engaged in reflective

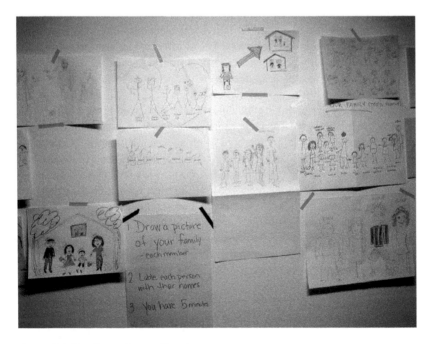

Figure 5.1 Family art therapy directive

dialogues that examined institutional programming and support for families affected by autism. To achieve these objectives, guided by the Museo ICO and cultural center hablarenarte in Madrid, together with three participating families from Spain, we all first visited professionals working in the education and access departments of select major museums of Madrid. We were given presentations by museum education and access department staff at the Prado Museum of Madrid, the Reina Sofía Museum, and the Thyssen-Bornemisza National Museum of Madrid. Through these presentations, we learned about each museum's existing programs for children and adults with disabilities and mental illness. All participants from both countries were able to exchange ideas and information on existing resources and to express their thoughts about the areas that need improvement to support families affected by autism. Two of the remaining three days focused on guided visits for learning about other various access-related resources or issues in Madrid. On these days, we also visited other cultural institutions such as hablarenarte, as well as the contemporary art and cultural programming center Matadero Madrid. Matadero is a unique, community-based cultural platform, a lively space at the service of creative processes, participatory artistic training, and dialogue between the various forms of creative arts, including music and literature. With the team of U.S. museum art therapists, and museum staff and parents from both countries, we observed programming and methods used by teaching artists and professionals working with individuals with autism and other diverse abilities in one of the buildings in the grounds of Matadero's large campus. The methods that were being used in the programming for individuals with disabilities and mental illness were open-studio-like, with a facilitator offering guidance, materials, and ongoing positive support and encouragement for the successful work of artists on their various projects. Matadero presented as one of the most interesting cultural centers with its numerous buildings spread over a vast campus and specific cultural programming for different age groups and populations being offered in each building. The large campus grounds were remarkably inclusive and designed to integrate populations of all ages and abilities in the pedestrianized grounds. On the last day of the retreat, the entire team of parents and professionals was invited to the U.S. Embassy in Madrid for a 2-hour meeting with the council and the team (2013). The meeting included a discussion of program goals, challenges, and community building, as well as heartfelt personal stories shared by parents about the importance of institutional partnerships of this kind for their children and themselves. This retreat resulted in a productive exchange between professionals from these cultural institutions and families, allowing everyone to learn about available programming in their respective countries.

Subsequently, a few months after the U.S. team's visit to Madrid, during their visit to the United States, parents from Spain came together to learn about the existing museum-based programs offered to students with autism in New York public schools, family programs, as well as Queens Museum's bimonthly open art studios for young adults with autism ages 17–24. In addition to visiting and developing programming in other cultural institutions in the area, participants had the opportunity to visit the partnering institution – the Queens Museum or Museo ICO, respectively. Delegates from both countries met in person to discuss important questions and issues raised by the program, such as various needs of families with children with autism and how a museum can help support those needs. During this site visit, the delegates learned first-hand about trends in autism services and lifestyles that are both unique to a setting and universal. Using the visit to discuss resources and spark public awareness, delegates also spent time with each respective institution's proven cultural partners to witness the greatest variety in access programming. For instance, Museo ICO participants visited museums in New York City, and Queens Museum's participants visited Asociación Argadini, a Spanish autism parents organization that has specific programs for visiting museums called "hablando con los museos," during which they invite their participants to give tours for their families.

By forming a group through these projects, parents in Spain learned how to create a network or community with each other and with U.S. parents to update and support one another. They were encouraged to share with a larger community of families through the access to cultural institutions' program participants. As noted, the initial retreat was followed by the Spanish team's visit to New York and after that, for 1 year, monthly workshops in each country, which were connected via Skype.

During these art therapy sessions, parents at the Queens Museum and parents at Museo ICO communicated via Skype to exchange information and learn from one another, contributing to the dialogue for change. Participants observed sessions via Skype during which they learned about autism goals developed by the community and curriculum plans in action. Parents also used information on education standards such as project-based learning, developmental stages of children, and how to use arts for social goals, occupational therapy needs, and social-emotional support. In addition to learning and exchange in real-time Skype sessions, parents also recorded and posted videos online for families who are unable to visit either museum. These activities created a forum where parents could engage in distance learning by observing recorded programs in the art studios and later receive opportunities to connect with participants and community-based partners. Moreover, these videos were coupled with an array of materials and resources that parents would be able to use as they participated at home with their children. A final visit of selected participants from each team to the other country took place at the end of the 1-year project.

Results

By forming a binational network of parent advocates, the emPower Parents program was initiated to work with parents on creating and using tools to request stronger programming for the inclusion of their children's different learning and expression styles in community programs. Parents who participated in the process of experimenting and being engaged in the creation of the best programming for their child with autism later engaged in the next level of participation, which was direct advocacy. Participating simultaneously in emPower Parents training and emPower Parents sessions, a practical application opportunity that put the project in action, placed program design and delivery into the parents' hands. This was already showing how they were evolving to emerge as new leaders by taking action to learn first and then participating in planning and facilitating workshop sessions, reflection, and action again. As noted before, taking place both at the Queens Museum and Museo ICO, the project was made up of six sets of parents in each location who were interested in having active leadership roles in the project.

Within the cycle of PAR (action, reflection, action), the results of the initial retreat and training led to action being taken where parents were co-leaders for a total of seven sessions. These included one opening information session and six sessions of direct contact with children. Parent participants engaged in a yearlong leadership opportunity that included active participation in the three areas of the program: session design and instruction, travel and conference, dissemination and advocacy.

The emPower Parents' initial training sessions for parents provided a place to practice those skills, the same opportunity that is given to new museum educators seeking to serve children with autism in museums' family programs. Parents gradually transitioned from observing to assisting, co-leading, and leading the family art sessions. The sessions in New York and Madrid happened simultaneously, in the morning in New York and in the afternoons in Madrid, allowing participants to connect virtually and share their artworks via Skype at the end of the sessions.

Session Design and Instruction

During the seven sessions of the project, participants trained with a staff of educators with a range of expertise as they learned how to design their own tools and curriculum for programming that targeted autism. The Queens Museum's participants used the current educator development tools, which were usually targeted at new educators and other professionals seeking to gain skills to better serve their community with autism. Instead, the parents used the tools and contributed as educators. Museo ICO's participating parents exchanged session experiences via Skype as well as using on-site training for their own learning. Parents from both countries contributed their recommendations for visual supports, providing positive behavior support, and identifying goals for each session.

Once parents had participated in these training sessions, they observed live sessions at the Queens Museum and live sessions of family programs through hablarenarte at Museo ICO. They were then invited to co-lead individual sessions of these family programs, as well as assist in documenting their own experiences through video and photography.

Assessment and Multiplying Community Art Programming

The Art*Access* art therapy program staff documented evidence that the emPower Parents project had strengthened the leadership skills of families affected by autism. Parents used the videos and photographs of sessions to critique and assess the progress of their own sessions. In addition, these firsthand experiences would become useful for the dissemination of community art programming for parents in various locations. The emPower Parents participants from both the Queens Museum and Museo ICO used this project as a means of further assessing their work through learning by doing. The project provided our staff and parent educators with a deeper understanding of their core knowledge that then helped them transform and improve their practice.

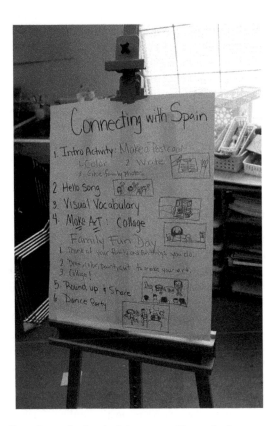

Figure 5.2 Outline of a session's schedule prepared by co-leaders

During art sessions, parents took on various roles including: (1.) two co-leaders; (2.) two facilitators who defined the goals of the sessions, making sure the group was following the outline (Figure 5.2) and providing overall direction in a clear, straightforward manner, and were responsible for group cohesion, pacing, and clear communication; (3.) a videographer, who collected videos of the sessions and interviewed students and parents for research and blog dissemination; (4.) a photographer, who took photographs to be disseminated online and to be used in group activities, such as researching images for the visual vocabulary, a printed tool used in sessions; and (5.) a communications coordinator who was responsible for connecting families in partner programs and managing the ArtPals exchange, a blog forum created for the collaboration where families could create artworks, exchange them via email or upload, and respond to another family's artwork by adding to the image creatively, facilitating a conversation through art that is inclusive for all children with autism, even those who are nonverbal.

Throughout the year, participants visited existing access programs at other cultural institutions, observing a range of the best practices for engaging children with autism and leading up to picking a partner institution of their choice to collaborate with to provide programming for families with autism. This endeavor included training other professionals and parents to independently use cultural institutions for the learning goals specific to each child.

The EmPower Parents program also gave parents a platform for sharing and practicing the leadership skills required for developing a network of parents in the community. For example, at the end of the 1-year project, one parent from the emPower Parents team in Queens, New York, created her own art program at the Queens Museum, Creative Spectrum, using the Art*Access* studio for her ongoing monthly sessions. She was able to coordinate other new parents and volunteers and lead a successful workshop on a monthly basis.

Dissemination and Advocacy

Throughout the emPower Parents training program, the participants at both the Queens Museum and Museo ICO created and developed a blog for dissemination of the lessons learned and personal reflections from participants. Through the blog, participants shared creative interventions with a larger community, including resources that have worked at home, in the community, and in the sessions they led during the emPower Parents project. Videos from the programs were shared on the blog in addition to existing resources. As our participants discovered and worked with new resources and tools, they were able to write blog posts or share images about them. The larger community that discovered the blog could also contribute, sharing their own personal stories. The rules for the blog were specified to all contributors, including privacy policies and safety recommendations when posting online. Such rules existed so that parents would not share their last names, addresses, or the schools their children were attending. Additional recommendations included making blogs visual, allowing visitors to the site that do not speak the language of the post to be able to understand the content via digital storytelling. Finally, through the blog, all visitors were encouraged to participate as ArtPals.

Discussion

A community of practice is based on joint learning rather than reified tasks that begin and end (Wenger, 1998). This was mostly visible from the beginning in that the emPower Parents participants from the museum who had been part of Museum Explorers Club family art therapy program for over 2 years had been serving as advisors to the program's autism initiatives and contributed to forming the model for the autism programming. They were given the opportunity to contribute more actively through the emPower Parents project. Similarly, participants in the Museo ICO and hablarenarte programs were informing the group of parents in Spain who were increasingly working with hablarenarte to share and collect resources.

Besides the training around the interdisciplinary work of museum art therapy, with the programming and workshops that took place over monthly sessions, parents practiced a variety of skills helpful in determining the best type of programming for their children, which included gaining the perspective of being a family art workshop facilitator and the understanding of how to develop and use visual supports by learning about and utilizing positive behavior support strategies.

Creative arts therapists share a universal language and they will find many opportunities for international and cross-cultural communication (McNiff, 2009). Specific art objects are tangible meeting points (McNiff, 2009), and the emPower Parents sessions were structured around those meeting points, evolving through the artistic processes that were happening simultaneously in New York and Madrid. Various cultural groups tend to similarly correspond in approaches to sharing feelings and discussing their group process (McNiff, 2009). This similarity was visible in sessions where families from two countries were sharing and discussing their processes during monthly sessions. Art therapy practice as it is being developed in the United States reflected characteristics of cross-cultural interchangeability (McNiff, 2009).

The art therapy practitioner will recognize the factual necessities that will determine the next steps. By abandoning styles of being that are purely ego-dominated, the nomadic subjectivity (Reyhani Ghadim, 2020) allows us to enter into relationships with an openness to understanding something new (Watkins, M. & Shulman, H. 2008). This attempt to change may lead to redefining the enterprise or adding elements to the repertoire of the practice (Wenger, 1998). The art therapist at the museum may engage in a nonhierarchical relationship of exchange with the community through participatory projects involving visitors and communities outside the museum, including interstate or international projects. The co-participants expressed the benefits of using the arts to shape the growth of the participatory project, surfacing important knowledge from which they developed networks for change. Working at an international level allows art therapy to maintain its flexibility and expand its community-based orientation.

The participatory project initiated the forming of new communities in which information could feed us and provide us with new knowledge and insight. If we are able to become a community, we will engage in civic discourse and conversations about how we expect the world to be and how we can strive to navigate it better (Carr, 2011). The participatory project opened a space for us in which we used the arts to inform us in ways that would have been impossible if we had been limited to discussions. Through art sessions, participant parents took on the role of leadership and practiced self-reflection through "learning by doing."

Summary

This chapter described a participatory project that was a result of inclusion and a vision of openness, making critical reflection an essential part of the role of the socially engaged art therapist's journey within community-based settings. This collaborative project was made possible owing to a partnership with not-for-profit organizations in the United States and Spain and six families in the U.S. and six families in Spain with one or more child(ren) with autism spectrum disorders. The cross-cultural initiative aimed to create change in intercultural programming structures to create, reinforce, and improve group workshops, dynamics, and facilitation with families affected by autism, and to empower parents to become leaders. It also aimed for art therapists and museum professionals to become involved in civic engagement in support of community-based programming. The outcome and participant feedback demonstrated that the binational participatory project strengthened the professional and personal development of professionals and participants, which in turn multiplied impacts on their communities.

References

Carr, D. (2011). *Open conversations, public learning in libraries and museums.* ABC-CLIO.

Eisner, E. W. (2012). *The arts and the creation of mind.* Yale University Press.

Elmendorf, D. (2010). Minding our P's through Q's: Addressing possibilities and precautions of community work through new questions, *Art Therapy: Journal of the American Art Therapy Association, 27*(1), 40–43, doi:10.1080/07421656.2010.101 29564

Freire, P. (1998). *Pedagogy of freedom, ethics, democracy, and civic courage.* Lanham, MD: Rowman & Littlefield.

hablarenarte. (2012). About us. www.hablarenarte.com/en/quienessomos/

Keenan, M., Dillenburger, K., Rottgers, H. R., Dounavi, K., Jonsdotir, S. L., Moderato, P., Schenk, J. J. A. M., Virues-Ortega, J. Roll-Petterson, L. R., & Martin, N. (2015). Autism and ABA: The gulf between North America and Europe. *Review Journal of Autism and Developmental Disorders, 2*, 167–183. https://rdcu.be/cbMxt

Kapitan, L. (2010). *An introduction to art therapy research.* Routledge.

Kapitan, L., Litell, M., & Torres, A. (2011) Creative art therapy in a community's participatory research and social transformation. *Art Therapy: Journal of the American Art Therapy Association, 28*(2), 64–73. doi:10.1080/07421656.2011.578238

McLaughlin, J. (2017). Why model autism programs are rare in public schools. Retrieved from: www.spectrumnews.org/opinion/viewpoint/model-autism-programs-rare-public-schools/

McNiff, S. (2009) Cross-cultural psychotherapy and art. *Art Therapy: Journal of the American Art Therapy Association, 26*(3), 100–106. doi:10.1080/07421656.2009.1 0129379

Moon, B. L.(2003). Art as a Witness to Our Times, *Art Therapy: Journal of the American Art Therapy Association,* 20:3, 173–176, DOI: 10.1080/07421656.2003.10129572

Peacock, K. (2012). Museum education and art therapy: Exploring an innovative partnership. *Art Therapy: Journal of the American Art Therapy Association, 29*(3), 133–137. doi:10.1080/07421656.2012.701604

Reyhani Dejkameh, M. & Shipps, R. (2019). From Please Touch to ArtAccess: The expansion of a museum-based art therapy program. *Art Therapy, 35*(4), 211–217. doi:10.1080/07421656.2018.1540821

Reyhani Ghadim, M. (2020). Nomadic art therapy: A contemporary epistemology for reconstructed practice. *Art Therapy.* doi:10.1080/07421656.2020.1746617

Think Spain. (2012). Autism affects one in 300 children in Spain. Retrieved from: www. thinkspain.com/news-spain/21002/autism-affects-one-in-300-children-in-spain

United States Embassy – Spain. (2013). News and events, Museum Connect, October 7, 2013. Retrieved from: http://madrid.usembassy.gov/news/events/events2013b/connect2013.html

Watkins, M. & Shulman, H. (2008). *Toward psychologies of liberation, critical theory and practice in psychology and the human sciences.* Palgrave Macmillan.

Wenger, E. (1998). *Communities of practice, learning, meaning, and identity.* Cambridge University Press.

6 Collaborating Organizations Help Interns Light Up the Panorama of the City of New York

Vida Sabbaghi

COPE NYC (Creative Opportunities Promoting Equality New York City) is a cultural arts organization directed by Vida Sabbaghi that collaborates with other organizations on local, national, and international projects. It believes in bringing people of diverse backgrounds together in safe spaces to discover their commonalities and differences. COPE NYC fosters creativity in its community projects, which include local and international artist residencies, traveling exhibitions, art education programs, and fashion shows. Its innovative programs connect student artists and art educators with commercial artists, galleries, and museums. When the dynamic, moving parts of academia, the art world, and the community come together, they create a vibrant collaboration.

In 2014, COPE NYC formed a partnership with the Queens Museum Department of Education's Art*Access* program. Art*Access* is internationally recognized for its programs for diverse populations. Instead of teaching artists, the art tour and art-making sessions are led by art therapists who design art experiences connected to the museum's exhibitions that promote the appreciation and enjoyment of art and enhance quality of life. Art*Access* has grown through the intersection of art therapy and art appreciation.

COPE NYC and Art*Access* are partners in using rhizomatic approach. Art*Access* welcomes teaching artists to tailor customized workshops to meet the needs of specific populations with diverse intellectual, emotional, and physical abilities. They scaffold the students' skills to reach higher goals and expectations. The 2018 internship program, which included high school students on the autism spectrum, a student with fluctuating mood, and young adults from a day rehabilitation center, is an exemplary model showing how partnerships among cultural institutions can create more effective outcomes for inclusive, accessible programs. "Art has special significance to . . . students with varying needs . . . because it helps develop interest, is therapeutic, and students may be misjudged if their creative talents are not considered" (Cromarty, 2017). Drawing from each organization's resources and strengths creates more productive outcomes for the populations they serve. In this chapter, I will discuss how COPE NYC collaborated with Art*Access* to customize internships for a specific cohort. I will start with a summary of the internship project and go on to explain how the 40 hours of preparation unfolded.

DOI: 10.4324/9781003014386-6

A Summary of the Panorama Tour Internship Project

Through the Rosemary Kennedy VSA Initiative, Art*Access* and COPE NYC educators prepared young adults, including those on the autism spectrum, to work as museum interns. They learned about the mission of the museum; the history of its prized exhibit, the Panorama of the City of New York; how to greet visitors; and how to answer questions about New York City.

Museum educators modified their professional development methods to meet the needs of the interns who learned about the Panorama through digital presentations, handouts, and tours. They worked in teams in preparation for engaging visitors for each borough and practiced dialogues in their own distinct style. On the day of the rehearsal for a tour visit, when a group of 20 students and their teachers came to each intern's station, some interns shared the many facts they had memorized, while others preferred to use a visual thinking strategy (Yenawine, 2013), asking visitors – "What do you see?"

The COPE NYC interns and the Queens Museum interns dressed professionally as they prepared to give a tour of the Panorama. On April 12, 2018, for the first time since its inception in 1964, the Panorama of the City of New

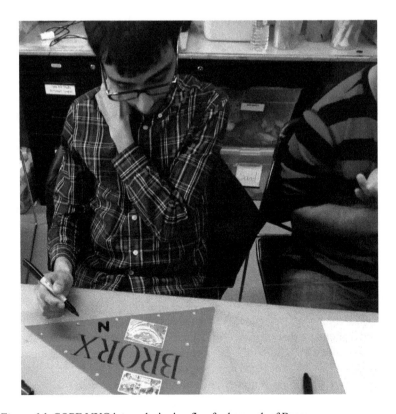

Figure 6.1 COPE NYC intern designing flag for borough of Bronx

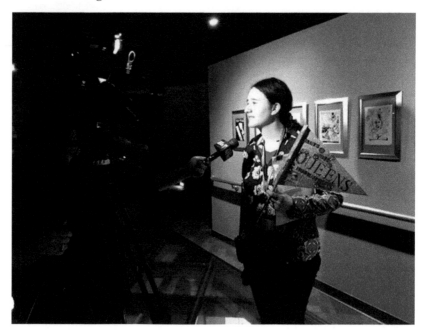

Figure 6.2 Intern interviewed by New York1

York tour was led by COPE NYC and Art*Access* student interns, with varying intellectual abilities, for a visiting group of high school students who also had varying abilities. The interns in-training created flags to hold when stationed next to a designated borough (Figure 6.1). The flags had text spelling out each borough and imagery of iconic landmarks.

The use of a flag provided a tangible support system which they relied on as a visual tool to reinforce what they learned, a physical aid to support them standing next to the boroughs, and text to support their presentation. The interns were excited and a little nervous about giving a tour. They had diffi-culty projecting their voices when practicing in a noisy, resonant environment. Adjustable headsets to amplify their voices made all the difference; they gave the interns the confidence they needed to do a great job, even when they were interviewed by NY1 about the tours they were facilitating (Figure 6.2).

Queens Museum Art Therapy Programs

Piloted in 1983 as Please Touch, to provide art education for people with vis-ual impairments, Art*Access* grew into a nationally replicated model designed to allow audiences of all abilities to enjoy a personal connection to art and cultural institutions. For three decades, each year, the Queens Museum pro-vided unique programs for thousands of children and adults with varying physical, emotional, behavioral, and cognitive abilities across the New York City area.

At the time of this project, Art*Access* programs were designed and led by full-time and part-time licensed art therapists. Art*Access* also partnered with various organizations that provide creative services for diverse populations. One of these organizations was COPE NYC, which had collaborated with Art-*Access* for 7 years through various satellite and on-site programs.

Rosemary Kennedy VSA Internship Initiative

In 2018, COPE NYC worked with the museum's art therapy program and its contractor, VSA, an international organization on arts and disability. Through the VSA Rosemary Kennedy Internship Initiative, students and young adults living with disabilities who have an interest in the arts, arts education, and arts administration are provided with hands-on experiential professional skill development opportunities (VSA, 2020)

Queens Museum is well known for its openness to the community. It is located on the site of the 1964 World's Fair in Corona Park. The Mets' Citi Field, the USTA Billy Jean King Tennis Center, and the New York Hall of Science are within walking distance. Local residents fill the park with food stands, ball games, ice skating, picnics, and family gatherings. The museum makes an extra effort to make the local community feel welcome with engaging outdoor play- or arts-based activities for children.

Art*Access* and COPE NYC strive to be accessible and inclusive for all populations. Both are inspired by educational theorist Viktor Lowenfeld's idea of meeting each individual and scaffolding his or her skills to higher goals (1953). In this case, museum art therapists and COPE NYC educators prepared a group of high school students on the spectrum and young adults enrolled in day rehabilitation services to be interns. They learned about the mission of the museum, the role of the museum's staff, and the history of the Panorama of the City of New York. The group also learned how to greet visitors and how to answer questions about NYC. They learned about the Panorama of the City of New York through digital presentations, handouts, and tours. They worked in teams for each borough and prepared dialogues in their own distinct style.

Emotional Support for Interns

The COPE NYC interns were paired with Art*Access* graduate art therapy program interns as an emotional support system. They wore identical ID badges. Both groups appreciated the pairing as they carried out several sessions rehearsing the procedure for facilitating tours for visitors to the museum. Visitors welcomed the interns' interacting and practicing, which included introducing themselves and giving an inquiry-based tour of the Panorama of the City of New York.

Learning the Roles of the Museum Staff

COPE NYC educators, and the student interns and young adults, began the internship program by visiting and learning about the museum exhibits and educational programs as a research organization. COPE NYC viewed the interns' roles as researchers of the museum. The interns learned about the museum's mission to serve as an educational institution and learned to connect their exhibits to the borough of Queens, the most ethnically diverse place in the world, where residents speak over 800 different languages (Lubin, 2017).

Focal Point of Internship: The Panorama
of the City Of New York

The Panorama of the City of New York, a three-dimensional model of NYC and its five boroughs that is one of the permanent exhibits at the Queens Museum, was the main focus of this internship. The Panorama was created by urban developer and World's Fair president Robert Moses for the 1964 World's Fair. In this scale model, where 1 inch equals 100 feet, the Statue of Liberty with its base is $3\frac{1}{4}$ inches tall. The Empire State Building is 15 inches tall. The total area of the five boroughs is more than 9,000 square feet.

Interns learned once or twice a week, over a course of a semester, (1.) how to research information; (2.) how to facilitate tours of the Panorama and (3.) how to lead art-making workshops connected to the Panorama for their peers and teachers alongside museum art therapists and interns.

Working with Interns to Learn to Lead
a Tour and a Workshop

Starting points for learning about the museum model included questions such as: What is a museum? What kinds of careers are available at a museum?

Coupled with digital presentations and inquiry-based sessions about the museum, its permanent and temporary exhibits, and the roles of the museum staff, we also carried out in-person introductions with museum professionals working in various departments in different capacities. Before we made the formal introductions of the interns to the museum professionals, we had a session around the importance of social etiquette in a professional environment being an essential part of internship. Interns learned that the dynamics involved in social interaction in the workplace are different from other societal relationships such as familial and casual relationships.

The internship involved learning about the five boroughs through (1.) digital presentations that clearly defined the roles of the interns and introduced the different staff in the museum, with focus on the Education Department; and (2.) hands-on instruction about leading a tour, planning a trip for peers and teachers, and applying sustainable methods while planning art-making workshop projects.

Paperwork and Journals

As an orientation, interns filled out paperwork for Art*Access* museum intern IDs. This was a great way to show COPE NYC interns they were part of and contributing members of the museum. Interns received journals to write and draw reflections of their experiences as researchers for the museum. Studies suggest:

> The internship can be a unique opportunity from which the student can learn about the nature of a particular job, career, organization or industry, and most importantly, themselves. One way to successfully capture this experience and extract additional meaning from it, is by keeping a journal of the internship experience. Keeping a journal develops an active and reflective learning posture rather than merely a passive one, and thus aids in grasping more of what the internship experience has to offer.
>
> (Laker, 2005, p. 63)

A Multitier Platform to Connect with the Panorama of the City of New York

As the entrance to the Panorama of the City of New York is dark, and some areas of the walkway have glass, it was necessary to practice adjustments and get acclimated to this unique environment in which a narrow walkway surrounds the monumental model of New York City. A typical day for interns was as follows:

1. Walk-through rehearsal
2. Discussion of how they interpret cities
3. PowerPoint presentations that emphasized the definition and role of the interns as researchers
4. Learning about museum resources with emphasis on the Education Department
5. Digital presentation of the history of the Panorama of the City of New York

Reinforcement of the same materials is important, especially for short-term memory.

Flags and Fun Facts

One of the ways we were able to reinforce the five boroughs' fun facts and highlights was for the interns to create flags for each borough. The flags were created with wooden dowels and stiff poster paper in the classic triangular shape found in many flags. The words and iconic symbols on the flags contained the information the interns needed for the tour. For example, on the Bronx flag, highlights included the Bronx Zoo and Yankee Stadium. On the Brooklyn flag, there were Nathan's Hotdogs and Coney Island. The flag's tactile nature also became a valuable support, boosting the interns' confidence as well as providing a colorful, fun way to greet and lead the crowd. The flags, with text that spelled out each borough, became a tangible support system which they relied on as a visual tool to reinforce what they learned, and a physical aid to support them standing next to the boroughs.

Amplify Your Voice

It was empowering to see the COPE NYC interns practice the tour. Each rehearsal was unique. Having the interns stationed as teams beside each borough proved effective. When they were engaged and their interest was sustained, they never wanted to stop practicing. The interns did have difficulty projecting their voices in a noisy environment during several practice walk throughs at the Panorama. To help amplify their voices, we bought headsets. The use of headsets created a more satisfying experience for interns and for visitors: it dramatically improved wider audience appeal through enjoyment-based education. It offered visitors better experiences with stories that connected people to objects, collections, galleries, and spaces. The acoustic challenges with simultaneous tours make headsets a great investment.

As the interns shared their thoughts about using the headsets, BT said: "JM, now you have headsets give it a try!" JM said: "I got this; I'm ready; I really like the headsets; I'm really happy." The fun, playful, interactive use of flags and headsets was like a game.

> A lot of studies have proven that the form of interactive games . . . has a good effect on children with autism . . . Reinforcement Learning (RL) for children with ASD, which has five interactive subgames . . . is necessary to establish and maintain compelling interactions in therapeutic process.
>
> (Li et al., 2019)

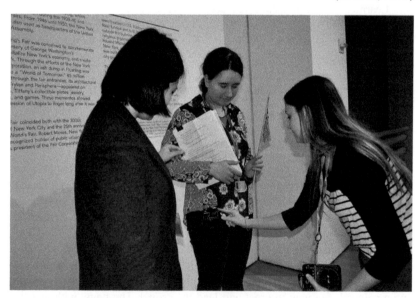

Figure 6.3 Adjusting headset to lead tour of the Panorama of the City of New York

The headsets were inexpensive and battery-operated, with FM radio. They amplified the interns' voices enough with volume controls (Figure 6.3). The range fit the needs of the interns who were giving the tour of the Panorama of the City of New York. We believe use of headsets for visitors taking tours of the exhibits are extremely helpful, especially in shared spaces found in museums where multiple tours and visitors are quite normal. We hope this practice will be used more often in the near future.

Working with Students with IEPs

Digital presentations became a valuable source of collective research. We were able to look at presentations and discuss the Panorama among ourselves. Interns were in a relaxed environment and shared their own associations with New York City's five boroughs. Previous observations of internships suggest interns with IEPs (individualized education programs), including those on the autism spectrum, are not given digital presentations as might usually be given to interns without IEPs. Providing a well-designed presentation for any cohort enrolled in an internship can be a dialogic tool, especially, in reinforcing their roles, the institution's mission, personal exchanges and dialogues, how to welcome visitors, and how to make introductions.

Visiting Other Cultural Institutions

The interns visited other cultural art institutions as researchers. They visited the Brooklyn Museum and the New York City creative reuse center, Materials for the Arts (MFTA). Interns can learn about each other while visiting other cultural organizations to learn about their mission and methodologies, and their education departments. Approaching the interns' experience with the idea that cultural institutions offer resources of information to learn from provides interns with a broader space for intellectual reflection and discussion among their peers. And they provide immeasurable opportunities for new ways of thinking about philosophy and practice, such as using touchable objects related to exhibits, which I will discuss later in the chapter.

When we organized the interns' visit to the Brooklyn Museum, we met with one of the museum's access educators who gave a tour of the museum, including the various entryways such as stairs and elevators.

The access educator asked which exhibit the interns would enjoy the most by providing a handful of choices. Prior to the visit, the Brooklyn Museum access educator emailed us a customized handout for the interns to review. It was good to have the information formatted in a way that would be helpful for individuals with varying intellectual abilities. Studies suggest that a cyclical relationship between visiting a museum and viewing its website can be rewarding. "The past few decades have witnessed unprecedented changes with respect to the use of museum information resources – changes that have resulted in new levels of access and new forms of interactivity for museum professionals and museum visitors" (Besser, 1997; Knell, 2003).

In recent years, we have seen steps towards customized museum access information available on digital platforms. This kind of support which helps us become familiar with a new environment before going there is a great way to scaffold one's ability to feel comfortable and to acclimate to a new situation. Educational theorist Lev Vygotsky defines the zone of proximal development as "the distance between the actual developmental level as determined by independent problem solving and the level of potential development as determined through problem solving under adult guidance or in collaboration with more capable peers" (Vygotsky, 1978, p. 86).

Brooklyn Museum, a larger museum with a different mission and larger archives, has more opportunities to give visitors objects, including artifacts, for integrated hands-on activities. Access to the conservation and restoration departments provides a more in-depth insight into the science of conservation, providing different ways of seeing and interpreting the work. Although the Queens Museum had a smaller range of resources, some artifacts were available, allowing integration of hands-on activities, especially connected to its permanent exhibits. But it did not have the wide range of replicas provided by the curatorial department necessary for interactive exhibits. However, for years, the art therapy program created tactile models for select exhibit articles to be used in their sessions with various populations. Many visitors, especially those with children, have come to expect interactive elements in museums. The Queens Museum does have a large collection of souvenirs from the 1939 and 1964 World's Fairs that would be ideal for hands-on activities. After visiting the Brooklyn Museum conservation and restoration departments, the interns had many questions. Exposure to another institution demonstrated the importance of a pluralistic approach rather than a single one.

How can the Queens Museum integrate interactive and participatory elements that relate to conservation and restoration, like the Brooklyn Museum does? Do other museums have internship programs for individuals with autism or other developmental differences? One of the interns opened up and told us he was also an intern at the Lincoln Center with its access program. It was rewarding to hear about the intern's experience in another institution, and it demonstrated he was comfortable enough to share this experience.

Trip to Materials for the Arts

The MFTA education coordinator provided us with a digital introduction before we went to the facility. All the digital information about the Brooklyn Museum and the MFTA, and their websites proved beneficial. "These changes have manifested most clearly in the relationships between museums, museum websites, and museum visitors" (Müller & World Institute for Development Economics Research, 2002, p. 338). Interns arrived at MFTA and were greeted by an educator who led the group up to the MFTA studio. Prior to the visit, the MFTA educator requested that each intern bring a recycled item for greater connectivity. After the interns shared their recycled items, a discussion ensued about how they might apply creative reuse techniques to the object they brought. They brainstormed and then went to the recycling area where materials were categorized. As the teams already had workshop plans, they had ideas about where to get the materials to best suit the workshop they will design. They were encouraged to touch the materials and to touch the artworks that used creative reuse techniques. The art materials gave them ideas for developing a workshop in connection with the tour of the Panorama.

Both Art*Access* art therapy interns and COPE NYC interns were able to go to MFTA together because their schedules aligned. For the Brooklyn Museum trip, only the COPE NYC interns were able to commit. It was difficult to coordinate both cohorts because everyone had very different course and work schedules. When Art*Access* interns rotated, it was confusing for some of the COPE NYC interns to understand. This was actually a positive challenge; it was great for preparedness training for transitioning to professional and career worlds, as colleagues, managers, and directors can change in a work environment.

The interns gathered information and collected and sorted materials for planning a museum workshop connected to the Panorama tour for their peers and teachers. They also needed materials for a workshop for a COPE NYC intergenerational group of more than 25 individuals with varying intellectual abilities.

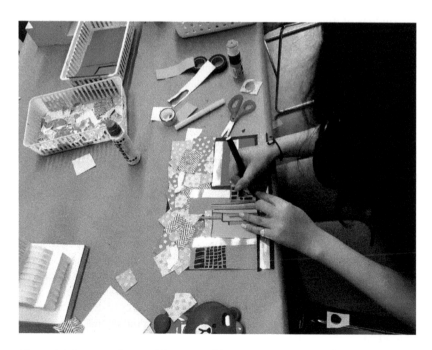

Figure 6.4 Intern at Queens Museum making a cityscape post-visit at Materials for the Arts

Materials for the Arts is a treasure for schools, nonprofits, and other cultural institutions. Donors from various organizations make MFTA a vital means for art teachers to be able to source materials to meet their curriculum needs (Figure 6.4). MFTA encourages art teachers to integrate materials for sustainable, recyclable, and/or, adaptive reuse projects into their lesson plans. The students incorporated the idea of "flags" inspired by a t-shirt exhibition at the Queens Museum.

Before they left, they also gathered materials for the culminating event workshops – paper-based collage cityscapes – popular workshops used in connection with the Panorama.

Day of the Tour

Two to three interns stood near each borough of the Panorama. One intern held the flag of the borough and welcomed visitors with some information about the borough. Each intern at the borough station would be able to help answer visitors' questions. A group of more than 20 students and their teachers came to the interns-in-training stations, next to each of the five boroughs. Some interns preferred to share many facts; others preferred to use a visual thinking strategy methodology.

Visual Thinking Strategy is a widely used

> educational non-profit that trains educators in schools, museums, and institutions of higher education to use a student-centered facilitation method and can create inclusive discussions. Their intensive professional development programs provide individuals with the tools to become skilled facilitators of complex conversations. VTS['s] . . . accessible classroom curricula are supportive of critical thinking, visual literacy, communication, and collaboration skills. Instead of providing content knowledge of an exhibition, they develop inquiry-based questions to ask the visitor.
>
> (VTS, n.d.)

An Art*Access* graduate art therapy intern's notes on the April 12 event encapsulate how most of us felt on the day when interns led the tour: "Today was a successful day on all parts. It is clear that there was much excitement and anticipation over the upcoming tour to be led by the interns." There were many aspects of preparation that I believe went into making the tour a success.

The interns were aided by multiple objects and technologies. To start, headsets and mics were key components in the success of the tour. For those who had soft voices or shy demeanors, the headsets were a major factor in contributing to their confidence and ability to project their voices and be heard. They were also very conscientious and were able to refrain from fidgeting or touching the buttons on the temperamental headsets. I had thought that this might be a problem, as the headsets have the potential to emit loud, disruptive, grating screeches.

I was glad that this did not occur and that the headsets functioned as needed. The interns were also aided by the flags they crafted. These flags were instrumental to the confidence and comfort of the interns. The borough flags were also a source of conversation and a way to introduce the topic to be discussed and viewed. They served as visual cues to the interns and the tour group themselves. The interns were also able to access their clipboards of information in case they needed guidance, clues, and reminders of the information they needed to know.

Lastly, the interns were aided by their own enthusiasm and eagerness to practice and guide a group of their peers. The tour went smoothly, and everyone enjoyed the cityscape directive that ensued.

Interns also suggested that the group should have been divided in half for the tours and studio workshop. The tour group was large, but that added to the excitement of the activity. The studio was much too crowded, but everyone participated and had a good time.

We all felt that the tour was a great success. The adjustable headsets used to amplify the interns' voices helped give them the confidence they needed. This rewarding experience was true to the Rosemary Kennedy VSA Initiative, which promotes opportunities for young adults with diverse abilities to work with cultural arts institutions for career development.

Museum art therapists and COPE NYC interns learned so much while working together. They learned about each other's interests. One intern loved to cook. So, on the last day, she taught everyone how to design cupcakes instead of buying snacks.

This is an important model of what COPE NYC does – listen to the cohort it is working with and provide opportunities for its members to share their skills by integrating them into the program. The curriculum of life is different for each student and always intersects with the learner's experience in school (Rolling, 2006). Interns received certificates for their commitment to be researchers at the museum. They provided invaluable and critical insights into how museum art therapists and COPE NYC can make their methodologies more effective for people with diverse backgrounds and abilities.

Conclusion

COPE NYC believes in fostering motivation and well-being for participants; creating opportunities for integration for people with different mental and physical abilities; and extending dialogue across distinct communities while promoting the formation of new knowledge and continued social interaction through the arts. Interdisciplinary art projects can be instrumental in fostering diversity by offering more visibility to communities not formerly engaged in the arts and a continuum of greater integration among contributing and exhibiting artists who have varying intellectual, physical, and mental abilities. This approach, using authentic real-life training, moves away from past training models, as interns are creating a scheduled program for a museum tour and workshop for the Education Department. In *Art as Experience*, Dewey suggested that art is unable to divest itself from the meanings of the past and should be present in all educational activities in the humanities (2009).

COPE NYC's mission to bridge communities was successfully achieved. The COPE NYC interns worked with museum art therapists in planning activities. They worked hard to prepare for the tour of the Panorama and they were very happy with the great job they did. They took pride in welcoming their peers and teachers for the tour of the Panorama, followed by a workshop connected to the tour. COPE NYC and the museum art therapists hoped they were laying the ground work for similar internship and training projects that would result in hiring individuals for paid positions in cultural institutions and other organizations.

References

Besser, H. (1997). The transformation of the museum and the way its perceived. In K. Jones-Garmil (Ed.), *The wired museum: Emerging technology and changing paradigms* (153–170). Washington, D.C.: American Association of Museums.

Cromarty, E. (2017). An educational historical narrative study of visualization in the progressive art pedagogy of Lowenfeld. ProQuest. Retrieved from: www.proquest.com/en-US/products/dissertations/individuals.shtml

Dewey, J. (2009). *Art as experience*. Perigee Books.

Knell, S. (2003). The shape of things to come: Museums in the technological landscape. *Museum and Society, 1*(3), 132–146.

Laker, D. R. (2005). Using journaling to extract greater meaning from the internship experience. *Journal of College Teaching & Learning, 2*(2), 63–71.

Lowenfeld, V. (1953). *Creative and mental growth*. Macmillan.

Lubin, G. (2017, February 15). Queens has more languages than anywhere in the world – here's where they're found. Retrieved December 07, 2020, from www.businessinsider.com/queens-languages-map-2017-2

Müller, P., & World Institute for Development Economics Research. (2002). Internet use in transition economies: Economic and institutional determinants. Helsinki: United Nations University, World Institute for Development Economics Research.

Rolling, J. H. (2006). Who is at the city gates? A surreptitious approach to curriculum-making in art education, *Art Education, 59*(6), 40–46.

VSA. (2020). The Kennedy Center. www.kennedy-center.org/education/vsa/

VTS. (n.d.). About us. Retrieved from: vtshome.org/about

Vygotsky, L. (1978). *Mind in society: The development of higher psychological processes*. Harvard University Press.

Yenawine, P. (2013). *Visual thinking strategies: Using art to deepen learning across school disciplines*. Harvard Education Press.

7 ARTogether

A Possibility of Therapeutically Informed Programming in a Museum Setting

Sarah Pousty

Introduction

Creating art and viewing art have the potential to provide a level of healing. The artist identity by its very nature can be a direct challenge to dominant culture and the status quo, and the work of artists can be a tool for guiding conversations about pushing boundaries and disrupting systems. Museums hold a place in our society for displaying, collecting, and storing art and art objects and, in turn, they play a role in holding space for the experience of artmaking and viewing. I have memories of experiencing certain pieces of art for the first time in a museum setting. As a young person trying to connect the different layers of my identity, I remember seeing work by contemporary artists such as Shirin Neshat, Louise Bourgeois, Lee Bontecou, Kara Walker, and Emily Jacir that helped me feel connected to something larger than myself. Their work presented me with images that spoke to me, challenged me, and helped me feel seen. Viewing their work in a museum setting added a significant level of importance and grandness to both the work I was viewing and how I viewed myself. Later, as I began to reconnect with my Iranian heritage, I would visit museums such as the Metropolitan Museum of Art (MET) in New York exclusively to see the Persian miniatures collection and Persian carpets. As my family is unable to return to Iran, it felt bittersweet to go to the MET and connect with these works and objects. In recent years, I have come to reflect on these experiences and how they informed my desire to work in museums.

While my reflections have led me to hold that museums can be a place of healing, access, and representation, I've simultaneously realized how they uphold narratives of colonialism and white supremacy. I have come to better understand how museums serve as a microcosm of the macrocosm: institutions with histories rooted in upholding the status of the wealthy and reflecting the values of white dominant culture (Robinson, 2017).

Currently, a significant number of museum workers, primarily education and frontline staff who represent the most diverse workers in museum institutions, have lost their jobs in the wake of the COVID-19 pandemic (Dávila, 2020). A museum as endowed as the Museum of Modern Art in New York laid off its entire freelance education staff through a single email, with no promise of return to work, stating, "It will be months, if not years, before we anticipate returning

DOI: 10.4324/9781003014386-7

to budget and operations levels to require educator services" (De Liscia, 2020). With the termination of educator contracts come the termination of community partnerships built over significant periods of time and the abrupt ending of relationships with New Yorkers who might not interact with the museum otherwise. This includes people who are experiencing homelessness, undocumented minors, people with disabilities, seniors, and court-involved youth (Steinhauer, 2020). Small and unendowed museums such as the Children's Museum of the Arts (CMA) made similar cuts, also citing challenges related to COVID-19. These cuts included ending its sponsorship of the ARTogether program, which will be the focus of this chapter. As Kerry Downey, an artist and MoMA Community Programs educator points out, "Educators were laid off at the moment NYC most urgently needed us. NYC communities did not disappear when the museum was closed" (Downey, 2020).

Amid months of quarantine because of the COVID-19 pandemic came the uprisings across the United States and around the world in response to the police murder of George Floyd in Minneapolis. Mass protests took place within all 50 states, with people demanding that Black Lives Matter. Many museums were quick to make statements of solidarity with the Black community and the protesters, publicly claiming on social media and on their landing pages that each museum was committed to fighting systemic racism. It is hard to trust these messages while the same museums simultaneously laid off their most diverse and lowest paid staff and dismantled programs that primarily serve historically marginalized communities.

I wonder how we can uplift the reason therapeutically informed work should exist in the museum space while holding institutions accountable to combat systemic racism. Arts leader and curator Yesomi Umolu (2020) outlines *"15 Points Museums Must Understand to Dismantle Structural Injustice"* and states, "Museums have long positioned their values and activities as apolitical acts of civic benevolence without probing their own proximity to power" (p. 2). Perhaps we begin by refusing to accept that museums are apolitical spaces, and, in order for deeper healing to occur there, museums must acknowledge and reckon with their own histories and positions of power.

Reflective Practice

As facilitators, we hold power and authority in our role, creating a power imbalance between us and the people we work with. Dr. Kenneth Hardy (2001) describes the tasks of the privileged and emphasizes impact over intent. It is important for us to understand our own position and role in the systems we work within as a way to actively reduce harm in these systems. In *Cultural Humility in Art Therapy*, Dr. Louvenia C. Jackson (2020) describes a lifelong reflective practice for developing "a worldview with integrity and respect for oneself and those one works with" (p. 19). In her chapter focusing on approaches to social justice she states:

> Social change begins with cultural humility, which is fostered in the knowing of self. When practicing social change, art therapists must be mindful

to understand their own values and not impose them on others, lest these values become another form of oppression.

(p. 117)

Having a reflective practice can serve as a guide for better understanding our own nuanced identities, what brought us to this work, and the impact our identities have on our practice. Reflection can be used to confront how we might uphold oppressive patterns in our work, inform accountability, and lead us to develop ways to actively shift power to the people we work with. The families I have worked with through my therapeutic practice predominately identify as Black, Latinx, and Chinese, from communities that have been historically under-resourced. As a light-skinned, first-generation U.S.-born Iranian in an upwardly mobile family, I recognize that I hold relative race and class privilege. I share this to acknowledge my position: where I stand in this work and the place I write from.

I have worked in New York City museum settings since 2003 and chose to pursue a degree in art therapy with the purpose of returning to the museum space to create therapeutically informed programming. In 2010, when I began to develop ARTogether with CMA, I was also working as a facilitator of art therapy-informed groups at the Queens Museum of Art and as an art therapist in a milieu setting, supporting the healing process of survivors of domestic violence. In this milieu, we worked from a team approach and operated within a trauma-informed and anti-racist framework. Race and power analysis were considered in every piece of our work with families, in our therapeutic interventions, and in our interpersonal interactions. This work continues to create shifts in me on every level, always revealing more work to be done. My learning, unlearning, and mentorship that began in the milieu inform how I practice my museum-based facilitation and the way ARTogether was developed.

In this chapter, I will be recounting the ARTogether program at the Children's Museum of the Arts from 2010 to 2020 as a case study of the possibility of creating therapeutically informed programming in a museum setting. I will describe how ARTogether was developed, our theoretical approach, the program's structure, and the program's suggested best practices. At the end of each section I will discuss the work presented through a social justice lens and use reflection as a tool to explore possibilities that were not realized through our program. My intention is to both uplift and interrogate the work we were able to build over 10 years and to offer the whole of our work, as I understand it at this moment, to inform future programs.

How ARTogether Developed

ARTogether explored this question: *How can a community arts program support the needs of families navigating the New York City child welfare system?* The CMA began considering this question in 2009 through a partnership with a local foster care agency. In this partnership, a professional artist who is also an experienced teaching artist and I, a trained art therapist, co-facilitated two multifamily groups at the agency. Each group met for six sessions. Group participants were families experiencing court-ordered separation and who had weekly mandatory visits scheduled at the agency. Supervising agency workers were present during group sessions, though they did not engage in the co-facilitation process.

The teaching artist and I developed each session to include artmaking directives that created opportunities for family members to collaborate and share their individual skills and interests. Together, they created a collaborative family shield with a symbolic crest and a quilt with patches representing family members' strengths and passions. We co-facilitated the group with a focus on community building by opening each session with a brief check-in or ice-breaker exercise and ending each session with an opportunity to share about the artwork created. During the artmaking portion of the session, we would walk around the space, connecting with each family individually to provide support when needed. After each group, the teaching artist and I would take time and care to reflect on the session. These debriefings would then influence our next session planning and ongoing co-facilitation practice.

Each program cycle culminated with a private celebration at the museum. The artwork made during the group sessions was displayed in the museum the evening of the event, and participating families enjoyed the offerings of the museum space. The attending agency workers observed and commented on the increase in ease when the families were sharing time at the museum as compared with at the agency. As facilitators, we also observed that the families appeared excited by the museum's play spaces and overall were more relaxed than they were during visits at the agency.

Around the same time, the museum learned of the Providence Children's Museum's Families Together program developed by Heidi Brinig. Families Together has been active since 1991 and is a nationally recognized therapeutic visit program for court-separated families in the Rhode Island child welfare system. The program is led and facilitated by a team of clinicians who are museum staff. The museum partners directly with Rhode Island's Department of Children, Youth, and Families, providing families with positive visitation experiences at the museum (Families Together Toolkit, 2006). CMA was inspired by the work of Families Together and the potential for children's museums to fill a gap of providing a natural, family-focused setting for families in foster care to engage in court-ordered visitation.

Upon researching the NYC child welfare system, consulting with the Families Together program, and speaking with a range of stakeholders, CMA became more familiar with the systems, policies, and potential partners involved with developing a museum-based visit program. The museum enlisted me to bring my art therapy training and experience to develop a program model centering the specific needs and strengths of families navigating the NYC child welfare system. In 2010, the museum received funding to pilot the ARTogether program, and we began to actively create a model of practice that developed over time.

2010–20

ARTogether at CMA became a community-based family support program that worked with families navigating the New York City child welfare system. ARTogether supported participating families by providing opportunities to have court-ordered visits and shared family time in a museum space that is specifically designed to support family engagement.

ARTogether worked with families receiving foster care services or preventive services, recently reunified families, families in kinship care, and families in the process of adoption. The ARTogether program paired participating families with a clinically trained facilitator who provided individualized support during scheduled museum visits (Pousty, 2020).

ARTogether was not a therapy program, nor was it a substitute for clinical therapy services. Our program was a community-based, therapeutically informed support program. We worked in partnership with a range of social service providers who were often a family's social worker and/or supported the family with direct therapeutic services. Our program built strong relationships over time with agencies across NYC's five boroughs, and continuous outreach was important, as there was regular turnover in the role of the workers we partnered with the most. ARTogether connected with referring workers and agencies through open house sessions and professional development opportunities that occurred both at the museum and in an agency setting. These opportunities allowed us to build relationships with providers by exchanging best practices, sharing awareness about our program's offerings, and regularly revisiting the question of how the museum can serve as a resource for families involved in the child welfare system (Pousty, 2020).

Discussion and Reflection

Research suggests that family visitation is the primary way that families remain connected and attachment relationships are supported during foster care separation (Mallon & Leashore, 2002). Family visitation is also linked to less time in foster care and better outcomes for children (Nesmith, 2015). Additionally, the quality of shared time during visits is regarded by family courts as an important factor toward a family's readiness for reunification. However, resources to support family visitation are typically limited, with visits taking place in agency office settings, where there are few supports for engagement and families may be reminded of the events that led them to enter the system. By partnering with social service agencies, ARTogether created an opportunity for family visits to shift away from agency settings to the museum space, which, as shared above, is intentionally designed and programmed to support family engagement. In our model, we were able to (1.) improve the quality and consistency of family visits; (2.) provide opportunity and support for families to practice skills developed in therapy, parenting classes, and groups in a natural community setting; and (3.) connect families to the larger cultural

continuum by engaging in artmaking, art viewing, imaginary play, and social-
izing in the community space of the museum (Pousty, 2020).

In 2010, when we began this work, the shift from the agency to the museum,
from my perspective, appeared to be a significant and transformative shift into
a more community-centered care practice. The agencies we partnered with
reflected a similar reaction and excitement for the program we were building. However, the word *community* needed to be looked at more closely, as
the participating families did not live in the West SoHo neighborhood of the
museum. By 2014, we recognized that the location of the museum was a barrier for many families, and we expanded our offerings to include the option of
facilitators working with families within the agency setting and in more local
community spaces, such as libraries. During the last 5 years of the program,
I became more aware of the cultural work and the spaces that are created in communities by its members. Looking to the future, I am interested in ways that
these cultural spaces, which are truly community-based and representative of
their populations, might be creating care practices and models that can inform
and lead the work being done to support families.

I also find myself reflecting on the question of whose voices were present
and whose voices were missing in the development of ARTogether. While we
built strong relationships with agencies and social service providers, I wonder
how our program and practice would have been impacted if we had created
similar partnerships with advocacy groups created and led by caregivers who
are most affected by the child welfare system. I believe the scope and perhaps even the purpose of our program would have shifted toward being more
inclusive and equitable if we had held listening sessions with caregivers where
they could voice how they could best be supported by CMA, both in the initial
development of our program and regularly thereafter when ARTogether was
active.

Theoretical Approach

ARTogether facilitators were clinically trained in the fields of art therapy, social
work, early intervention, and counseling (Pousty, 2020). Facilitators had prior
experience of using art viewing and artmaking in their work with families in
conjunction with their particular clinical training. Facilitators worked directly
with participating families, and each facilitator brought a unique set of skills,
insights, experiences, and creative possibility to the work. ARTogether facilitators came from diverse ethnic backgrounds in an attempt to reflect the families
in the program. This was intentional as it increased the possibility of pairing
families with a facilitator who could provide culturally competent support and,
when needed, bilingual support. Pairing families with a facilitator of a shared
background also had the potential to increase the family's ability to feel better
understood and more at ease to advocate for their needs (Pousty, 2020).

ARTogether used an interdisciplinary approach to support families on relational goals such as improving communication and improving parent–child

connection (López & Pousty, 2015; Pousty, 2020). Our approach combined best practice models from attachment research, community-based art therapy practice, and museum education.

Attachment Research

Attachment research informed how we worked with each family as a connected unit. We recognized that child welfare involvement had the potential to disrupt attachment relationships in a range of ways, including: through a precipitating event such as a child experiencing or witnessing abuse, neglect, or maltreatment involving a primary caretaker; through court-ordered separation as in the case of a family with a child living in foster care; and through the potentially harmful effects the system's approach to care can have on the life of the family it is meant to support and protect. Our approach was trauma-informed, and we recognized the researched benefits and protective factors of secure attachment and nurturing caregiver–child relationships (Bowlby, 1982; Siegel & Hartzell, 2003; Bryant, 2016; Chesmore et al., 2017). ARTogether supported familial bonds between children and the legal parent(s) being monitored by the child welfare system through shared creative experiences and individualized support that paralleled therapeutic parent–child dyad work (Proulx, 2003; Lieberman & Van Horn, 2008; Toth et al., 2013).

Community-based Art Therapy

Community-based art therapy informed how facilitators drew from their therapeutic training to provide support for participating families while recognizing that the purpose of the work in the community setting was to hold space for empowerment, reduction of stigma, nurturing connections between participants, and increased social inclusion (Hocoy, 2007; Ottemiller & Awais, 2016). This approach also allowed for skills that participating families were developing in therapy settings and psychoeducation groups (such as parenting groups) to be put into practice in the natural setting of the community, with the support of a trained facilitator if needed (López & Pousty, 2015). We recognized the significance of engaging in creative processes. The process of making art became an active way for families to connect through the collaboration, communication, and negotiation required when working together and/or alongside one another. Through making and viewing art, families were able to lead the exploration of their own personal narratives, curiosities, and togetherness. The concrete nature of a finished product could serve as a way to encapsulate shared creative experiences and maintain connection for families between visits, especially for families that were experiencing court-ordered separation.

The community-based art therapy model differed from clinical art therapy practice most clearly in the environment of the community setting and in its approach. ARTogether facilitators did not analyze artwork for diagnostic purposes, did not use artwork as means of exploring therapeutic material such as trauma, and did not use observations to pathologize. When therapeutic material did arise in the form of a metaphor in the artwork or artmaking process, facilitators maintained a role of being a witness and stayed present with what was being shared, ensuring that the participant was in the lead of their expression and creative exploration. If appropriate, for example, when a parent expressed a struggle to maintain their parental authority, a facilitator might develop a directive with a structure or particular material that would encourage increased success in this area. When participants initiated sharing therapeutic material directly, the facilitator would witness and acknowledge what was being said, support the family to remain in the current moment, and connect the family back to the partnering referring worker who would support the family to explore the material in the safety of a clinical space.

Museum Education

Museum education informed our belief that hosting family visits in the community space of the museum allows families to build a relationship with the museum space itself and offers the potential for families to independently utilize the museum as a resource for shared family engagement once they completed the ARTogether program. Lannes and Monsein Rhodes (2019) describe the potential for museums to serve as a "third place" or gathering place for different intersections of the community to engage together with a sense of communal belonging. Shifting family visits from the agency settings to the community setting of the museum has the potential to reduce stigma that families involved in the child welfare system might experience.

When considering a framework for exploring and viewing artwork, the program pulled from the research-based strategies of visual thinking strategies (VTS) developed by Abigail Housen and Philip Yenawine (López & Pousty, 2015; Dejkameh, Candiano, & Shipps, 2018). This model uses questions to draw from participants' own experiences and expertise to assign meaning and narrative to works of art, both in the gallery space of the museum and in the artwork created by participants. It is a success-based model that encourages cognitive thinking skills, curiosity, and respectful listening to multiple perspectives (López & Pousty, 2015). The VTS model for exploring artwork parallels the common practice of art therapists who support clients in assigning their own narratives and meaning to their finished artworks by asking open-ended questions about the work.

Discussion and Reflection

Understanding the oppressive patterns that exist within the child welfare system were important in informing our approach to working with families. In a data-filled report centering firsthand parent accounts, Lisa Sangoi and Movement for Family Power (2020) state, "The child welfare and foster system holds perhaps the greatest power a state can exercise over its people: the power to forcibly take children away from parents and permanently sever parent–child relationships" (p. 10). Children in foster care have experienced abuse, neglect, or maltreatment of some kind, as determined by a child welfare investigation that has the power to obtain a court order to separate families. Research suggests there are increased risks and negative outcomes for children removed from the home as compared with children of similar socio-economic background who remain in the home (Lawrence, Carlson, & Egeland, 2006; Sangoi & Movement for Family Power, 2020). As understanding of how traumatic the experience of separating children and families can be has become more recognized, the national trend since 2002 has moved to increasing preventive services instead of removal (Yaroni et al., 2014). However, by the end of 2016, there remained 437,465 children in care nationally (Child Welfare Information Gateway, 2018).

The criminalization of poverty and institutionalized racism critically dictate how the child welfare system functions. Sangoi and Movement for Family Power's report (2020) illustrates the ways low-income Black, American Indian, Latinx, and White mothers are targeted by the child welfare system, specifically around allegations of substance use. The authors point out how the system's "Focus on individual responsibility for alleged parenting failures completely ignore societal ills that often instigate involvement in the first place" (p. 6). Institutionalized racism is reflected in the disproportionality of Black-, American Indian-, and Latinx-identifying families in the system (Sangoi & Movement for Family Power, 2020). In her book *Shattered Bonds: The Color of Child Welfare*, Dorothy Roberts (2009) centers the voices of Black and African American mothers fighting to have their children returned to their care. Roberts connects the parent accounts to national data and research describing the additional challenges and mistreatment that Black and African American families face when navigating the system as compared with their non-Black counterparts. These inequalities reveal the influence of anti-Black racism and cultural bias on the child welfare system.

ARTogether's main premise was to support familial bonds between children and their legal parents while the relationship was being monitored by the NYC child welfare system. Our main tool to support a family to strengthen, repair, and/or maintain family connections was through shared creative experiences. The facilitation team influenced what the ARTogether program did through its practice of co-creating the work with participating families. Along with attempting to pair families with a facilitator who had a shared cultural and/or racial background, conversations about anti-racist and anti-oppressive practice began during the facilitator interview process. Potential ARTogether facilitators were asked about how they approach race, privilege, and power in their work. Interviewees were made aware that discussing these topics would be part of supervision. The need for supervision to be built into the ARTogether program came from my own early experiences while being the only person in the facilitator role and without case supervision. Within the co-construction of the supervisory relationship, we were able to reflect on our work with families, question cultural norms and norms of practice, and plan interventions that included accountability and disrupting oppressive patterns (Pousty, 2020).

In reflecting on the work in this section, I realized that we did not directly connect our work to a social justice-centered practice and pedagogy. While anti-racist and anti-oppressive practice informed the development, practice, and discussion of our work within the program, we did not center this approach outwardly – for example, in our printed materials, grant writing, or program descriptions. As can be seen in this section, anti-racist and anti-oppressive practice was not listed in our above theoretical approaches. I am curious about this omission and who it was for. In this current moment, I feel aware of the increase in open discussion and normalization of social justice-centered pedagogy and practice. This environment feels outwardly different from the environment in which we were building ARTogether, and I wonder how this shift in public discourse will influence the work to come.

Program Structure

Families were most often referred to ARTogether by a caseworker, social worker, therapist, attorney, or a parent advocate with whom they had a close relationship. ARTogether did not ask families or referring workers to share about the precipitating event that led the family into the child welfare system. We aimed to work with families in the present moment of their relationship and believed that it was the family's choice to share their story. This is often in contrast to the child welfare system, which expects families to repeat difficult stories despite the painful effect that this retelling might have (Pousty, 2020).

Once a family was accepted to ARTogether and paired with a facilitator, the next step in the process was to schedule an initial intake meeting before family visits began. This meeting took place at the museum and was attended by the referring worker, ARTogether facilitator, and participating caregiver. The purpose of the intake meeting was for the caregiver to travel to the museum, become familiar with the museum's offerings, and connect with their assigned facilitator in advance of coming to the space with their child. This experience was meant to affirm the caregiver's adult role and aimed to increase the caregiver's confidence to lead their child in the space when visits began. During the initial intake meeting, the visit schedule and individualized program goals were developed collaboratively. When appropriate, the family's current therapeutic goals were shared for the purpose of setting program goals that overlapped and supported the family's larger child welfare case. In this meeting, the caregiver would give consent for continued open communication between the worker, facilitator, and caregiver, allowing for progress to be shared and for overlapping support to be provided.

Each ARTogether visit was 2 hours long. CMA is a unique children's museum that focuses exclusively on art viewing and artmaking. The mission of the Children's Museum of the Arts is to introduce children and their families to the transformative power of the arts by providing opportunities to make art side by side with working artists (Children's Museum of the Arts, 2020). The museum has a large gallery space in the center that hosts rotating exhibitions throughout the year. Exhibits include works of contemporary art and, often, pieces from the museum's permanent collection of children's artworks from around the world. The museum has three main areas: a media lab, a fine art studio, and an early childhood studio. Each space offers programming that ranges from being self-guided, such as creating a drawing by looking at a still life, to artist-led workshops that are inspired by the current exhibition and the teaching artist's own area of expertise.

During a family visit, the ARTogether facilitator guided the family through the museum space and workshops for the first hour and facilitated a private artmaking experience with the family during the second hour. A typical ARTogether visit schedule was as follows:

- *Arrival* (15 minutes): Participating family checks in at front desk for museum entry stickers. Facilitator meets family in front and leads them to ARTogether family room for feelings check-in, review of rules set by family, and discussion of plan for public time.
- *Public museum time* (45 minutes): Participating family explores workshops and imaginary play spaces and views artwork in museum gallery space. Facilitator provides support as needed and pulls back when family displays ease and comfort navigating space independently.
- *Private artmaking time in ARTogether room* (30–45 minutes): Facilitator introduces artmaking directives that draw on family's interests. Projects are typically designed with the caregiver and/or entire family over the course of the program. Private-time projects allow for more intimate interactions. Examples of projects include stop-motion animation films, a family koi pond, a family meal sculpture, and family photo books.
- *Final museum exploration* (10 minutes): The family revisits a space they enjoyed or may save a particular part of the museum for this portion of the visit. Popular spaces are the museum's swirl chair studio or the museum's Quiet Room, which is also a book nook.
- *Final reflection and feelings check* (10 minutes): Family returns to the ARTogether room and reflects on the visit. A final feeling check-in is shared, and the next visit date is named.

Participating families experienced between 6 and 12 biweekly visits with their facilitator and, upon completing the program, received renewable museum membership. We did not track or record if families used their membership upon completing the program. Facilitators did remain in contact with families through our Aftercare program. Through Aftercare, we called to check in with families around how they were doing and offered to meet at the museum if they were interested in using their membership and wanted our support. We also talked with families about what types of resources they would like to connect with in their community and provided recommendations of cultural and community centers that were centrally located to where they live.

Lastly, as clinically trained professionals, ARTogether facilitators were able to provide reports of progress toward set goals and advocacy letters to family court with the consent and at the request of participating caregivers. Sometimes we observed big gestures; however, most often we witnessed the small gestures that collectively led to more connected relationships (López & Pousty, 2015). Our written reports highlighted families' strengths, attendance, affection, and shared creative experiences while in the program. We recognized that we were one piece of a participating family's support system and only a brief part of their journey as a family. We were focused on our role to support families in their goal of strengthening relationships in the moments that we shared with them.

Discussion and Reflection

Families were connected with us as ARTogether facilitators specifically because they were involved in the child welfare system. It was necessary for us to be aware of our association with this system, even when we did not share the values of the system. Themes of surveillance and control came up repeatedly in the child welfare system and echoed out into our work with families.

When I reflect on this section, I am reminded of the intentional ways that we designed ARTogether to reduce patterns of surveillance and control – for example, not asking families about what led them to being involved with the child welfare system and intentionally not tracking if families choose to use their membership of CMA. We had to return to these themes again and again to be able to make changes as our perspective on and understanding of patterns of harm grew over time. Reflection was a tool used to build understanding that led to concrete actions. In reflecting on surveillance, we considered and reconsidered how we discussed consent with families, how we shared progress about our work with families, and the language we used in our documentation. Reflecting on how control showed up in our practice guided us to consider how we were working to co-create art directives with participating families and if the family was in the lead of their own creative narrative. Reflecting on control also provided us with information about if and how we were holding space for families to express (directly or creatively) about mistrust of workers and the system without responding defensively.

In writing this section, my attention also comes back to the importance of cultural humility, the importance of building relationships with a foundation in knowing ourselves and seeing and being curious about the nuances of each family and family member we work with. Jackson (2020) explains, "Being open to other ways of knowing through art can allow for the individual or community to be viewed as rich experts and teachers on the context of their culture, avoiding 'isms' that cause stress in community life" (p. 26). Cultural humility combined with artmaking provides a path for holding complexity. Through this approach, we can hold our understanding of systems and the possible impact of systems on the families we work with while building a space where each participant is the expert on their own experiences.

Best Practices

The ARTogether model focused on supporting both the caregiver and child as they engaged with each other and continued to strengthen and/or repair their relationship. The following were the program's suggested best practices:

Praise

By providing praise and encouragement to children and parents, facilitators help families recognize the strengths of each family member. Facilitators model praise and work toward helping family members increase their ability to praise and point out each other's strengths. In a system that often focuses on what parents have done wrong or behaviors that need correcting, self-esteem and hope can be restored in families by highlighting nurturing qualities such as generosity, affection, help, confidence, bravery, and connectivity.

Balanced Support

Facilitators may serve as emotional, behavioral, and cultural translators between parent and child to increase mutual understanding. An example of this is helping a parent more accurately appraise their child's behavior by understanding how the behavior is related to their developmental level. Another example is verbalizing the intention behind a behavior. For example, a parent's frustration about the child not following directions can be reframed by the facilitator as the parent's emotional intention of wanting to see their child succeed and benefit from the activity.

Child-led Exploration

While parents set and maintain the visit structure, children lead the exploration and play in the museum. When parents follow their child's lead, they are able to learn about their child's interests and are encouraged to stay at their child's developmental level. Mirroring can be experienced as an affirmation and acknowledgment of attunement. Working alongside one another while creating artwork or engaging in side-by-side play can serve as a metaphor for mirroring and, as a result, strengthen familial bonds.

Strengthening the Parent's Identity as Caregiver

Parents with children in foster care often have limited access to their children's lives, as well as limited power to make decisions for their children while they are in care. This can deteriorate a parent's identity as the caregiver from the perspective of both the parent and the child. By supporting parents to lead activities, set limits, and engage independently with their children, facilitators send the message that they trust the parents' judgment and ability to care for their children. In turn, children witness their parents being treated with care and respect.

Modeling

As the ARTogether program takes place during public hours, participating families have the opportunity to observe and engage with other families visiting the museum. Facilitators might encourage parents to observe the behaviors of other children and reflect on what they notice. Parents are frequently surprised at how similar their child's behaviors are to those of their peers. Similarly, parents observe the ways other families interact, set limits, and manage difficult behavior. Then they reflect with the facilitator on techniques they may want to try or how they may have handled a situation differently.

Building Feeling Vocabulary

ARTogether facilitators begin and end each session with a "feeling check-in." Using a visual feeling chart, the facilitator supports family members as they practice both verbalizing their feelings and listening to each other's feelings without judgment or retaliation. When children share difficult emotions such as anger or sadness, they provide caregivers the opportunity to help them regulate their emotions or to bear witness to how they feel. Sharing feelings of love and happiness can provide an opportunity to verbalize how much a family enjoys being in each other's company (Pousty, 2020, pp. 274–275).

Discussion and Reflection

In the introduction to *The Revolution Will Not Be Funded*, Andrea Smith (2007) describes how the nonprofit industrial complex, "Promotes a social movement culture that is non-collaborative, narrowly focused, and competitive. . . . This culture prevents activists from having collaborative dialogues where we can honestly share our failures as well as our successes" (p. 10). Smith goes on to describe how focusing on and repeating what we have told funders is successful leads to inflexibility, which is counter to the creation of the flexible strategy that's needed in movements for social transformation (Smith, 2007).

This list of best practices was first written in 2015 when we created a PDF guide discussing the ARTogether model. This shareable PDF was both a public offering and teaching tool. These practices were never updated. I believe that the claiming of these practices in writing, sharing them publicly and with our funders, the positive feedback we received, and the culture of the nonprofit system we worked within all contributed to us being inflexible in the re-examining of this piece of our work.

Looking now, our lack of perspective is reflected in some of the language we used to talk about our practices and, inherently, in some of the best practices themselves. Most notable is the practice and description of *modeling*. We intentionally designed ARTogether to take place during public museum hours and within a community space of families who are experiencing moments of public joy and struggle in their ongoing caregiving/care-receiving experience. While this experience has the potential to reduce stigma and feelings of isolation for families affected by the child welfare system, it ignores the intersections of class and race that continue to be activated in museums that are reflective of dominant White culture. What are we saying to families of color when we hold whiteness up as a model or comparison? What are museum institutions saying when they sponsor programming for historically marginalized communities without actively shifting power and resources and without creating authentic representation within the museum space?

Yesomi Umolu (2020) warns against inclusion policies without change to the culture and institutional structure of the museum and names the task of this moment as, "uprooting weak foundations and rebuilding upon new healthy ones" (p. 3). Perhaps transformative programs that center social change, built with and for communities most affected, can be one part of Umolu's vision, one piece of the new, healthy museum foundation to come.

References

Bowlby, J. (1982). *Attachment and loss, vol. 1: Attachment.* New York, NY: Basic Books.

Bryant, R. A. (2016). Social attachments and traumatic stress. *European Journal of Psychotraumatology, 7.* https://doi.org/10.3402/ejpt.v7.29065

Chesmore, A. A., Weiler, L. M., Trump, L. J., Landers, A. L., & Taussig, H. N. (2017). Maltreated children in out-of-home care: The relation between attachment quality and internalizing symptoms. *Journal of Child and Family Studies, 26*(2), 381–392. https://doi/10.1007/s10826-016-0567-6

Children's Museum of the Arts. (2020) Mission statement. Retrieved on August 31, 2020 from: www.cmany.org/about/

Child Welfare Information Gateway. (2018). Foster care statistics 2016 [PDF file]. Retrieved from: www.childwelfare.gov/pubPDFs/foster.pdf

Dávila, A. (2020). In memoriam of the art world's romance with diversity. Hyperallergic. Retrieved from: https://hyperallergic.com/556290/in-memoriam-of-the-art-worlds-romance-with-diversity/

Dejkameh, M., Candiano, J., & Shipps, R. (2018). Paving new ways to exploration in cultural institutions: A gallery guide to inclusive art-based engagement in cultural institutions. Queens Museum of Art.

De Liscia, V. (2020). MoMA terminates all museum educator contracts. Hyperallergic. Retrieved from: https://hyperallergic.com/551571/moma-educator-contracts/

Downey, K. [kerrythat]. (2020, August 27). Today MoMA reopens without its educators [Instagram post]. Retrieved September 16, 2020, from: www.instagram.com/p/CEZaKUul3vs/

Families Together Toolkit. (2006). Families together toolkit [PDF File]. Retrieved from http://providencechildrensmuseum.org/wp-content/uploads/2020/07/FamiliesTogetherToolKit.pdf

Hardy, K. (2001). African American experience and the healing relationship. In D. Denborough (Ed.), *Family therapy: Exploring the field's past, present and possible futures*. Adelaide, Australia: Dulwich Centre. Retrieved from: https://dulwich-centre.com.au/articles-about-narrative-therapy/african-american- experience/

Hocoy, D. (2007). Art therapy as a tool for social change: A conceptual model. In F. Kaplan (Ed.), *Art therapy and social action* (21–39). Philadelphia, PA: Jessica Kingsley.

Jackson, L. C. (2020). *Cultural humility in art therapy.* Philadelphia & London: Jessica Kingsley.

Lannes, P., & Monsein Rhodes, L. (2019). Museums as allies: Mobilizing to address migration. *Journal of Museum Education, 44*(1), 4–12. https://doi.org/10.1080/1059 8650.2018.1563453

Lawrence, C., Carlson, E., & Egeland, B., (2006). The impact of foster care on development. *Development and Psychopathology, 18*(1), 57–76. https://doi.org/10.1017/ S0954579406060044

Lieberman, A. F., & Van Horn, P. (2008). *Psychotherapy with infants and young children: Repairing the effects of stress and trauma on early attachment.* New York, NY: Guilford Press.

López, M., & Pousty, S. (2015). ARTogether [PDF file]. Retrieved from https://cmany. org/wp-content/uploads/2017/01/ARTogether_V2_PDF-1-4.pdf

Mallon, C., & Leashore, B. (2002). Preface. *Child Welfare, 81*, 95–99.

Nesmith, A. (2015). Factors influencing the regularity of parental visits with children in foster care. *Child & Adolescent Social Work Journal, 32*(3), 219–228. https://doi. org/10.1007/s10560-014-0360-6

Ottemiller, D. D., & Awais, Y. (2016). A model for art therapists in community-based practice. *Art Therapy: Journal of the American Art Therapy Association, 33*(3), 144–150. https://doi.org/10.1080/07421656.2016.1199245

Pousty, S. (2020). ARTogether: Putting community at the center of family visits. In M. Berberian & B. Davis (Eds.), *Art therapy practice for resilient youth* (267–283). New York & London: Routledge.

Proulx, L. (2003). *Strengthening emotional ties through parent–child-dyad art therapy.* London: Jessica Kingsley.

Roberts, D. (2009). *Shattered bonds: The color of child welfare.* New York, NY: Basic Books.

Robinson, C. (2017). Editorial. *Journal of Museum Education, 42*(2), 99–101. https:// doi.org/10.1080/10598650.2017.1310485

Sangoi, L., & Movement for Family Power. (2020). "Whatever they do, I'm her comfort, I'm her protector": How the foster system has become ground zero for the U.S. drug war [PDF file]. Movement for Family Power. Retrieved from: https:// static1.squarespace.com/static/5be5ed0fd274cb7c8a5d0cba/t/5eead939ca509d4e 36a89277/1592449422870/MFP+Drug+War+Foster+System+Report.pdf

Siegel, D. J., & Hartzell, M. (2003). *Parenting from the inside out.* New York, NY: Penguin Random House.

Smith, A. (2007). Introduction: The revolution will not be funded. In Encite! (Ed.), *The revolution will not be funded* (1–18). Durham, NC, & London: Duke University Press.

Steinhauer, J. (2020). A crisis in community reach: MoMA's arts educators on the consequences of their contract cuts. *The Art Newspaper.* Retrieved from www. theartnewspaper.com/analysis/moma-cuts-art-educators-amid-funding-squeeze

Toth, S. L., Gravener-Davis, J., Guild, D. J., & Cicchetti, D. (2013). Relational interventions for child maltreatment: Past, present, and future perspectives. *Development and Psychopathology*, *25*(4), 1601–1617. https://doi.org/10.1017/S0954579413000795

Umolu, Y. (2020). On the limits of care and knowledge: 15 points museums must understand to dismantle structural injustice. *Artnet News*. Retrieved from: https://news.artnet.com/about/yesomi-umolu-1516

Yaroni, A., Shanahan, R., Rosenblum, R., & Ross, T. (2014). Innovation in NYC health and human services policy [PDF file]. Vera Institute of Justice. Retrieved from: www1.nyc.gov/assets/opportunity/pdf/policybriefs/child-welfare-brief.pdf

8 Museum of Fine Arts, Boston's Artful Healing

Putting the ART in Partnership

Alice Garfield

I check my list again, making sure I have the right room number. I don't hear voices, though the low mumble of a TV seeps through. Shifting my tray to free a gloved hand, I knock firmly on the wooden door. I think I hear someone respond, but just faintly. I push down the silver handle and enter, balancing my tray carefully. The first half of the room is dimly lit and uninhabited. I see an empty adjustable bed with side rails, an institutional blue faux-leather armchair, and an array of vacant ports and equipment on the walls, all partitioned off from the far side of the room by a patterned blue-and-white curtain hanging from a track in the ceiling. I walk past the end of the curtain and peer into the small pocket of room on the other side, brightly lit by the window at its far end. A young woman reclines in a bed just like the one I passed on my way in. Monitors behind her flash dimly with numbers and jagged lines. She has dark hair, and dark eyes that turn away from the TV. Her eyes widen in apprehension as she sees my yellow mask and gown. A woman sitting on a low padded bench under the window looks up from her phone. I pause just past the curtain, using my free hand to wave in what I hope is a reassuring manner. "Hi!" I begin, speaking loudly so I can be heard through my mask. "My name is Alice and I work at the Museum of Fine Arts. I brought an activity. Would you be interested in making some art today?"

The Museum of Fine Arts, Boston (MFA) has worked with hospitals and healthcare centers in the Boston area since 2007 to provide meaningful art engagement opportunities for individuals undergoing medical treatment. As the coordinator for the MFA's Artful Healing program, I have seen firsthand the positive influence that art and artmaking can have on wellness and healing, and the unique ways museums can facilitate this positive impact. Research has helped to confirm what arts and health professionals have witnessed and know to be true: art helps, heals, and holds us together in difficult times.

Art museums are not primarily considered a resource for health and wellness, but recent research supports that visiting an art museum or gallery can provide emotional and physical benefits. As Ioannides (2016) summarizes,

DOI: 10.4324/9781003014386-8

"museums enhance quality of life as well as facilitate the improvement of mental and physical health. Notably, people's well-being is enhanced if they engage with cultural collections and ideas in the company of other people" (p. 102). Many cultural institutions have begun to embrace new roles as facilitators of health and well-being for audiences as diverse as veterans (www.intrepidmuseum.org/veterans-and-military-families.aspx), adults with memory loss and dementia (www.americansforthearts.org/2019/05/15/museums-and-creative-aging), new mothers (https://breatheahr.org/melodies-for-mums/), children in the foster care system (www.local-level.org.uk/uploads/8/2/1/0/8210988/maclareportfinal.pdf), refugees (www.npr.org/2020/02/17/795920834/refugee-docents-help-bring-a-museums-global-collection-to-life), and more.

This chapter will focus on the partnership between MFA Artful Healing and Boston Children's Hospital (BCH), highlighting the ways in which these major Boston institutions have worked together to build a partnership that enriches the museum, the hospital, and broader Boston communities. Through this and other similar partnerships, BCH offers an outstanding patient experience, helping patients feel connected to the outside world while receiving top-quality medical care. The MFA is able to reach an audience beyond its walls by sharing its collections with those who may not feel the museum is a place for them.

Program Overview

The MFA Artful Healing program operates under the museum's Learning Department, alongside other programs labeled Community Arts. Artful Healing and other Community Arts programs focus on outreach and developing partnerships with community organizations. The mission of the Artful Healing program is to promote health, wellness, and healing through engagement with the MFA's collection and exhibitions, and to provide creative respite for children, teens, and families in medical settings. The Artful Healing program was inspired by the experience of an employee in the museum's Education Department who spent many hours in hospitals as a child watching her brother battle Burkitt's lymphoma. The MFA has established on-site workshops for children at BCH, Massachusetts General Hospital, and Dana-Farber Cancer Institute, with an additional partnership recently developed to provide artmaking workshops for adults receiving inpatient psychiatric treatment at Brigham and Women's Faulkner Hospital. Since 2007, the MFA Artful Healing program has reached over 10,000 participants. More than 5,000 of those participants have engaged in Artful Healing workshops at BCH.

What we aim to do through Artful Healing is to bring the museum experience into hospital settings and invite participants to visit the museum in person when they are able. Artful Healing educators facilitate this invitation by providing free museum passes to participants and their families, and scholarships to take studio art classes at the MFA. We receive numerous requests and inquiries about providing Artful Healing activities at new sites – both for additional sites within BCH and at other hospitals. The most significant challenge we have faced in expanding Artful Healing to meet this demand has been in securing sustainable funding for the program. Through generous donations from MFA patrons, we have been able to provide Artful Healing activities for free to our partner hospitals, though that is now changing out of necessity. Our programs at BCH remain free to the hospital and all participants, but we have forged new fee-for-service partnerships with partner hospitals that have secured grants or fundraised with their own generous donors.

MFA Artful Healing workshops at BCH are free to participants and occur at regularly scheduled times. Lessons are designed and taught by paid museum educators who have completed the hospital's volunteer training process. Educators also work closely with the museum's Accessibility Department, receiving accessibility training to expand their expertise in working with visitors and program participants with a wide range of physical, cognitive, and behavioral needs and abilities. Artful Healing educators design unique, engaging activities tailored to each location and population that they visit within the hospital, which can range from toddlers in a clinic waiting room to teens in the inpatient psychiatric unit. All activities use studio-quality, hospital-safe materials and encompass art techniques including, but not limited to, Chinese brush painting, Styrofoam printmaking, wire sculptures, painting on canvas, sculpting with clay, and embossing foil pendants. Each workshop has a central theme drawn from the MFA's collections and exhibitions. Museum educators begin each workshop with a presentation of images of artworks from the MFA collection, allowing participants an opportunity to "explore" the museum and connect with artworks spanning six continents and thousands of years of history.

In Artful Healing visits, images of artwork from the MFA provide artistic inspiration, but also serve as "third things" or intermediary objects that allow individuals to connect with something less personal than themselves. Writer and educator Parker Palmer describes the use of the "third thing" as a way to approach a difficult topic indirectly, thus making it less intimidating:

> We achieve *indirection* by exploring that topic metaphorically, via a poem, a story, a piece of music, or a work of art that embodies it. I call these embodiments "third things" because they represent neither the voice of the facilitator nor the voice of a participant. They have voices of their own, voices that tell the truth about a topic but, in the manner of metaphors, tell it on the slant. Mediated by a third thing, truth can emerge from, and return to, our awareness at whatever pace and depth we are able to handle – sometimes inwardly in silence, sometimes aloud in community – giving the shy soul the protective cover it needs.
>
> (Palmer, 2009, p. 92)

Looking at and making art can help individuals access and identify their emotions and can provide a safe space for participants to process difficult feelings.

As observed by Gelo, Klassen, and Gracely (2015),

> images of paintings may be used to facilitate conversation, rather than using direct questions about the patient's experience of illness and hospitalization. In this way, an image allows a patient to focus on something other than himself or herself and may stimulate thought. Frequently it is easier and less threatening for a patient to talk about an image, painting, photograph, or sculpture that captures his or her attention than to speak directly about fears, concerns, loneliness, and pain. Using images of artworks draws from narrative therapy and the process of externalization to express emotions (White & Epston, 1990).
>
> (p. 43)

The girl's tension melts away as she smiles and nods. The woman smiles too and gets up to help me adjust the bed and position a table over the girl's lap. I ask the girl her name, how old she is. She answers my questions (Leila, 10) but shakes her head when I ask if she's been to an art museum before. As I set down my tray, I explain a little more about the museum, showing the girl printed photos of paintings by Claude Monet, Vincent van Gogh, and Georgia O'Keeffe. I tell her I chose these artworks because all of the artists liked to paint landscapes near their homes. We discuss what "landscape" means, and what you might see in a landscape. I ask which of the paintings she likes best, and she instantly points to Vincent van Gogh's *Houses at Auvers*. An IV line trails from her raised hand.

"What do you like about it?" I ask, tilting the paper so I can see where she indicates.

"The clouds," she whispers, her fingers brushing across the top of the page. "The colors."

I point out how the clouds are made up of small blobs of paint, the way they blend into the sky, the wiggly outlines of the houses and trees. I ask if she wants to try making a painting of her own, and she nods enthusiastically. I show her the materials on the tray – watercolor paints, oil pastels, pencils, and heavy paper. I explain that if you start drawing with oil pastels first, you can paint on top with the watercolors and fill in big areas of color. She hesitates, unsure where to start. "Do you have an idea of what place you want to draw?" I ask.

"Mountains," she says softly, "and trees and flowers. And a sunrise." I suggest that she start with a pencil and lightly draw the areas she wants to be mountains, sky, and ground. She sketches hesitantly, but with deep concentration.

The woman – her mother, I learn – watches her daughter, intent on her work, and turns to me.

"Would it be alright if I take a shower?" she asks. I can see how tired she is, how stress and worry have settled in her shoulders.

"Of course," I say, "I'll stay with her while you do." She nods and turns to her daughter. She speaks to the girl in a language I don't understand, and Leila glances up and replies, wincing a little bit. The woman replies with sympathy in her voice, then steps into the small bathroom and closes the door. I settle into a chair next to the bed to talk with my young student.

"It hurts," she explains, sketching mountains in the background.

"That's no fun," I reply, shaking my head. "Does it hurt to draw?"

"No, no," she says, "I don't think about that now."

"What do you think about?" I ask, curious.

"That picture," she replies, nodding towards *Houses at Auvers*. "I would like to go there. It reminds me of my home."

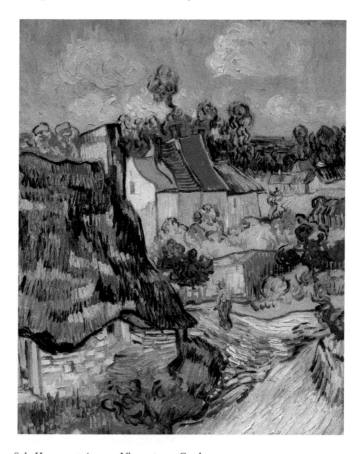

Figure 8.1 Houses at Auvers, Vincent van Gogh

Houses at Auvers, Vincent van Gogh (Dutch (worked in France), 1853–1890) 1890 Oil on canvas Bequest of John T. Spaulding Photograph © Museum of Fine Arts, Boston

Program Expansion

In 2007, the MFA and BCH partnered to provide Artful Healing workshops for patients and families in the hospital's Patient Entertainment Center. The partnership between the two institutions was prompted by the shared belief that art is a powerful tool that can aid families and children in difficult circumstances. By allowing children's imaginations to wander and families to simply have fun together, these workshops provide positive distractions resulting in beautiful works of art. Following the success of this program, the MFA's presence at BCH expanded to include workshops offered in hospital playrooms, family resource centers, group settings, and individual patient rooms.

In 2012, Artful Healing began working with BCH's inpatient psychiatric unit to offer a monthly group workshop for patients and staff. Existing Artful Healing activities had to be adjusted to meet the requirements of materials safety in a psychiatric setting, as some materials (foil, string, scissors, etc.) are restricted because patients could potentially use them to cause harm. The unit's staff members work with patients on developing positive coping mechanisms and behaviors, and Artful Healing educators have developed a variety of projects to support this positive growth, including collage, paper sculpture, printmaking, fashion design, and activities focusing on wellness themes including mindfulness, gratitude, and positive affirmations.

Our partnership with BCH has adapted and grown over a period of 13 years, most notably reflected in our participation numbers. During the first year Artful Healing workshops were offered in the Patient Entertainment Center at BCH, 200 patients participated over the course of ten visits during the year. In 2019, more than 600 participants engaged in Artful Healing programming during 61 visits made during the year. This growth and change reflect adjustments the MFA has made to Artful Healing programming in response to feedback from BCH staff. In 2012, BCH Child Life staff observed that their patient acuity was increasing and, while interest in artmaking remained high, they had a higher volume of patients who were unable to join in activities in public spaces owing to infection risks, mobility limitations, and pain. Artful Healing educators began making regular visits to inpatient floors and visiting patients in their rooms, bringing art inspiration and artmaking activities to those who needed them most.

Program Evaluation

Artful Healing staff and leadership have long been involved with local, regional, and national efforts to recognize the work of arts-in-health professionals and to advance the field. MFA staff have been involved with various professional arts in health organizations from the (now-defunct) Arts and Health Alliance to the Boston Arts Consortium for Health (BACH) and the National Organization for Arts in Health (NOAH). Through our work with NOAH and related organizations, we hope to contribute to the growing body of evidence-based arts in health practice.

Although Artful Healing workshops are not framed or evaluated as therapy programs, our observations and interactions with participants make it clear that looking at and making art are inherently therapeutic activities, especially for children and families enduring the stress of hospitalization. Research supports the positive impact of arts engagement on children's social and behavioral development (Fancourt & Steptoe, 2019), as well as its benefits in reducing anxiety (Sahiner & Bal, 2016) and increasing quality of life (Madden et al., 2010) for children undergoing hospitalization or surgery.

In 2013, the MFA hired an outside consultant to conduct an independent evaluation of participant experiences, outcomes, barriers, and improvements for Artful Healing at BCH. The evaluation included observations of programs, interviews, and focus groups with patients, parents/caregivers, hospital staff, and Artful Healing educators. Findings were "strikingly consistent across informant groups and hospital settings, and suggested core patterns of experience and positive outcomes that resonate closely with Artful Healing program goals" (Payne, 2014, p. 1). Engagement, enjoyment, social interaction, education, and access to art were identified as defining characteristics of the Artful Healing program. The evaluation found positive outcomes in all characteristic areas, including improved patient and caregiver well-being, increased effectiveness and job performance for hospital staff, and greater exposure to the arts for socio-economically disadvantaged patient populations.

Evaluation feedback from BCH consistently shows that our healthcare partners value the flexible, self-sufficient, and adaptable nature of Artful Healing programming and educators. BCH staff who work closely with Artful Healing have pointed to the flexibility of Artful Healing staff and programming as one of the most valuable parts of the program, noting that we have collectively tried several different approaches to working with patient and caregiver populations. Through our mutual willingness to try new ideas, we've found several that work best. From October 2016 through December 2017, Artful Healing educators made an extra monthly visit to the 9th- and 10th-floor inpatient units at BCH to work specifically with parents and caregivers of patients. We received some of our most heartfelt thanks and positive feedback from these visits but learned that caregivers were hesitant to leave children's rooms to complete an activity just for themselves. The low attendance for these visits prompted a meeting with BCH Child Life staff, who suggested moving our caregiver visits to the hospital's Hale Family Center for Families, where caregivers often wait before meetings with care teams, check emails on the center's computers, get information from the desk staff, or help themselves to free coffee. Our visits to the Hale Family Center are frequently attended by patients, siblings, and caregivers.

We talk about home, and about nature. She has finished her sketch and started to draw details: a field of flowers in the foreground, a stream flowing down from the distant mountains, leaves on the trees. She is telling me proudly that her art teacher taught her how to draw clouds, and demonstrating in white oil pastel, when a knock comes at the door and a woman in a yellow gown walks in. Her gown is covering blue hospital scrubs, and I can tell she is smiling underneath her mask. She speaks warmly, addresses Leila by name, asks how she's feeling.

"Where's mom?" the nurse asks, cheerily. The girl gestures towards the bathroom, intent on her work.

"She's just taking a shower," I reply, "do you need her?"

"No, I'll talk to her whenever she's done," she says, tapping at a keyboard under the flashing monitors. "We'll just get some vitals for now."

"Should I come back later?" I ask. She shakes her head.

"Oh no," she says, "it's great that you're here! You're keeping her busy. I'll work around you."

She bustles around the room, eyeing numbers on the monitor, asking questions and typing notes. The girl answers her questions quietly, focused on her artwork.

"What a beautiful drawing!" the nurse exclaims, her eyes crinkling in a smile above her mask as she adjusts a blue cuff around the girl's upper arm. The bathroom door opens and Leila's mother steps out, hair wet, dressed in the same clothes. The nurse greets her by name and asks how she's doing.

"I feel better now," the mother says, smiling.

"I'm glad!" the nurse responds, warmly. "I'm just getting some vitals right now, and then the doctor will come in a little bit to talk to you." Leila looks up at her mother, her eyes concerned, and asks what I can tell is a question. Her mother replies gently and turns to the nurse.

"She must wait for more pain medication, yes?" she asks. "The doctor said they changed her medication and she must wait to start the new one?" The nurse nods, confirming.

"Yes, I'm sorry – I know it hurts," she says to the girl, "but the new medicine will be better. You just have to be a little bit patient. We can give her ibuprofen in between," she says, turning to the mother. This information is translated to Leila through her mother, her response discussed and then translated back to the nurse:

"Yes, she will have that, please." The nurse leaves, saying she will be back soon, and that the doctor is coming. The girl's brow furrows as she returns to drawing, her expression anxious.

I show her the watercolor paints and brushes I've laid out on the tray and demonstrate how to paint on top of her drawing, how the oil pastels will resist the water and remain visible. She picks up a paintbrush and copies me, painting a blue wash across the top of her paper – the sky behind the mountains. Her white clouds float in the middle of the blue wash like islands. I hold up *Houses at Auvers*, and we look at the clouds again, how they melt into the sky. She uses a blue oil pastel to blend the edges of the clouds.

As she starts to paint in the mountains, three gowned people knock and enter the room. A tall woman introduces herself to us as the doctor and explains that the young man and woman with her are medical residents. I offer to come back later if they need to talk privately. My young student looks anxiously at her mother, then at me.

"No, we won't be a minute," says the doctor, "I want to check on a few things, and have a talk with Mom." I smile reassuringly at Leila, then lean down to straighten items on the tray in my lap, carefully looking away as the doctor reclines the hospital bed down and presses gently on Leila's abdomen. She asks the girl questions about her pain, and Leila answers, her voice tight. The doctor raises the bed back to a sitting position, then beckons Leila's mother and the residents to follow her as she walks past the curtain to the unoccupied half of the room. I can hear their voices but can only catch a few words of their conversation. The girl in the bed stares at the edge of the curtain, breathing fast.

"Are you okay?" I ask her. She shrugs stiffly, her voice coming out quiet and scratchy.

"It really hurts," she whispers. Tears well in her dark eyes and start to spill down her cheeks.

"Do you want to paint more? Or maybe not?" I ask, locating a small box of tissues on a countertop and offering them to her. She takes a tissue and wipes her eyes, sniffling.

"I want to finish my picture," she says. "I think I can do it." I nod and place the tray back in front of her. I hold up the image of van Gogh's painting.

"Let's look at this again first," I offer, "and see what else you might want to add to your picture." Her eyes sweep over the image, her attention drawn out of herself and into a countryside scene. She paints the mountains brown, with green trees and a blue river running down from a central valley. She draws the sun setting between the mountains in arcs of yellow and orange. She adds a pink house in the foreground, with dark wiggly edges like van Gogh's houses. She is starting to dot tiny flowers over the field next to the house when her mother pushes back the edge of the curtain and walks in, accompanied by the nurse from before. I didn't notice the doctor leave, or the nurse arrive. Leila looks up at her mother, smiling, her pain momentarily forgotten.

Special Considerations

For a program that consistently brings joy to participants, we do encounter our share of difficult and saddening experiences. One of the persistent difficulties of this work its unpredictability: we never know exactly who we'll be working with on a given day, and what their medical, physical, mental, neurological, and emotional needs and abilities are. Unpredictability is present in all aspects of our work, from how many participants we see during a given session to how long we can work with them and whether our visit will be interrupted by medical necessities. To address some of these uncertainties, we develop flexible and accessible art activities that can be adapted to meet a wide variety of needs and abilities and work closely with our participants to tailor the activity to them. We do also encounter situations that are emotionally difficult, especially when we connect with a participant who is experiencing pain and trauma. We never know if we will see a participant again, and sometimes we feel there is not enough we can do to help. The Artful Healing educators and I meet monthly to discuss these and other issues, and I consult with our hospital partners on ways to address some of the uncertainties we face.

Artful Healing educators are incorporated into the hospital's structure through the robust volunteer program, though we are self-maintained and directly communicate with Child Life staff to schedule and structure our visits. As hospital volunteers, we are bound by HIPAA and patient confidentiality laws, and we are trained to recognize the boundaries between what is necessary for us to know to fulfill our role and what information is not necessary. We sometimes need to ask about specific abilities, disabilities, mobility, and pain, where that information is important in providing the fullest possible art engagement experience, but a patient's diagnosis and prognosis are never necessary information. Despite this, our participants are human, as are we, and they seek human connection. Children in particular are eager to share stories about themselves and less aware of the boundaries that protect personal information. While they are absorbed in making art, participants often feel comfortable enough to share stories about traumatic injuries and illnesses, about deaths of family members and friends, about their struggles with mental illness or drug abuse. We report any concerning information to the relevant hospital staff for each unit and sometimes ask for guidance on how to manage difficult situations that arise. Our training recommends that we gently redirect these personal conversations, and we have all developed positive, respectful methods of guiding participants away from sharing personal information. One of the best ways I've found is to refocus on the artwork in front of them, grounding the conversation in concrete, present objects and events. Sometimes, though, the most helpful thing I can do is listen.

As the girl shows her mother her artwork, I ask if she's done painting and if she wants to display her artwork in her room. She nods, and we find a bare spot on the wall where I hang her painting up with loops of masking tape.

"Do you want to keep this?" I ask, holding out the printed copy of *Houses at Auvers*. She smiles and points to the wall next to her painting. I hang Vincent van Gogh's masterpiece next to hers.

I thank her for making art with me and offer them free passes to visit the museum, where they can see this painting and many others. They both thank me, and her mother takes two passes. I pick up the tray and leftover materials, leaving some extra blank paper and a pencil. I remove my gown, mask, and gloves near the door, then wave a final goodbye and exit the room. Outside, I rub my hands with sanitizer and carry the tray down the hall to clean my materials. As I wipe the paintbrushes and pencils with disinfecting wipes, I take a deep breath, and smile.

Artful Healing is supported by the June Nordblom Robinson Fund, Norman and Heewon Cerk, and Peter F. Kiely. With thanks also for the support of the Claudy family.

I would like to include my deep and heartfelt thanks to all the hospital staff, museum staff, donors, and participants I've worked with to build and maintain this wonderful program.

No real names are used.

References

Fancourt, D., & Steptoe, A. (2019). Effects of creativity on social and behavioral adjustment in 7- to 11-year-old children. *Annals of the New York Academy of Sciences, 1438*(1), 30–39. https://doi.org/10.1111/nyas.13944

Gelo, F., Klassen, A. C., & Gracely, E. (2014). Patient use of images of artworks to promote conversation and enhance coping with hospitalization. *Arts & Health, 7*(1), 42–53. doi:10.1080/17533015.2014.961492

Ioannides, E. (2016). Museums as therapeutic environments and the contribution of art therapy. *Museum International, 68*(3–4), 98–109. doi:10.1111/muse.12125

Madden, J. R., Mowry, P., Gao, D., Cullen, P. M., & Foreman, N. K. (2010). Creative arts therapy improves quality of life for pediatric brain tumor patients receiving outpatient chemotherapy. *Journal of Pediatric Oncology Nursing, 27*(3), 133–145. doi:10.1177/1043454209355452

Palmer, P. J. (2009). *A hidden wholeness: The journey toward an undivided life.* John Wiley.

Payne, J. (2014). Improving experience of care in hospital settings through engagement in the arts: An evaluation of the Museum of Fine Arts, Boston's Artful Healing program. Jessica Payne Consulting.

Sahiner, N. C., & Bal, M. D. (2016). The effects of three different distraction methods on pain and anxiety in children. *Journal of Child Health Care, 20*(3), 277–285. doi:10.1177/1367493515587062

9 People inside Museums

One Hands-on Artmaking Room in Context

Rachel Shipps

This chapter focuses on the ways in which art museums can be social and therapeutic spaces through incidental interaction and use of materials, and by promoting the feeling of agency. Visitors and their experiences are considered to be primary elements of public spaces in museums. Guiding this exploration is a commitment to the importance of museum access.

One important way in which museums promote well-being is by enabling individual agency and access to encounters with art and self-directed learning. Another consists of incidental opportunities for social connection. These two important elements, choice and interaction, are brought together in areas which are not uniformly present in art museums but are becoming increasingly visible: rooms that are directly adjacent to museum galleries designated as public areas may provide hands-on opportunities for exploring exhibitions.

Artmaking rooms adjacent to galleries have several evident strengths and hold the possibility of expanding visitors' experience of agency, qualitatively changing the focus of museum visits. In these spaces, multimodal interpretive materials and interventions are often made available. These may offer visitors multiple ways of experiencing museum exhibitions, as visitors can actively participate in a creative process that involves art as "a non-verbal medium for communication" (Silverman, 1989, p. 141). Such opportunities, in addition to providing multisensory means of engagement with the museum beyond the visual and textual, "can help activate, in particularly direct ways, the embodied ways of knowing that are so essential to aesthetic experience" (Hubard, 2007, p. 48). Through an overview of the conceptual setting and materials of one such piloted room, the MakeArt Lab at my workplace, San Francisco's Museum of Craft and Design, I examine opportunities for creative and physical access.

Situating Museums

In thinking through the physical space of museums, it is important to situate museums within their larger social context, which can be understood as a series of cultural holding containers. Visitors are held within a socially, intellectually, and aesthetically bounded gallery, which is held within the larger museum,

DOI: 10.4324/9781003014386–9

within the larger town or city, and finally within a civic and cultural regional or state structure. Each container is nestled within another like a set of matryoshka dolls. Educational and therapeutic groups that meet within the museum define another containing and supportive framework, which strongly shapes the experience of museum visits (Froggett & Trustram, 2014). Often, considering harmony and dissonance within this series of containing structures helps illuminate the nature of a museum and contextualize its construction and display of public space. That symbolic presentation is influential: "Museum and exhibition culture . . . can offer multiple narratives of meaning at a time when the metanarratives of modernity . . . have lost their persuasiveness" (Huyssen, quoted in Palmer, 2008, p. 59). These cultural layers of meaning influence the expected scripts, layout, and performances that take place within museums, including exhibition design, interpretation, and programs; these in turn can be used, expanded, and disrupted.

Some aspects of the museum space that guide visitor experience are what Charles Garoian has termed "performing the museum": conventions of movement, labeling, lighting, and temperature, and the visitor's knowledge of the museum workers' roles (Garoian, 2001, p. 247). Space and display, like exhibition objects themselves, are modes of expression of a museum's symbolic meaning and its social function. One frequently performed function of the modern museum is that of maintaining a physical and often symbolic distance between visitors and gallery objects. However, these divisions are not innate to artistic display or to museums themselves; vision was not always so culturally prioritized as a tool for perception and understanding. In some European museums in the 17th and 18th centuries, touch was considered to convey more reliable information and access to objects than perhaps any other sense. While "the eye might be deceived by skillful artifice" (Classen, 2007, p. 901), touch was seen as straightforward and immediate, a means of gathering fact and evidence, with the ability to "create physical and emotional connections with other peoples and places" (Classen, 2007, p. 903). Other senses such as scent were also considered in museum visits as part of a holistic appreciation of an object. Vision became the primary mode of museum presentation in part to preserve materials and accord with then-developing scientific priorities, but also as part of an institutional tension in museums as they became more public. Classen notes that

> it may have been as much the desire of the elite to prevent the lower classes from showing disrespect towards the cultural and political authority museum pieces were seen to represent, as the modern emphasis on conservation and the development of more visually-oriented models of science and aesthetics, that resulted in the non-visual senses being almost entirely shut out of the museum by the mid-nineteenth century.
> (Classen, 2007, p. 908)

If new scientific principles, vision, concerns of conservation, and social constraint had restricted the "social prestige, of touching with one's own hands artifacts and artworks" (Classen, 2007, p. 903), these factors also affected public access to "acquiring and conveying an air of cultural authority" (Classen, 2007, p. 897). Within a museum setting providing only visual information, the nominally public setting is sometimes at odds with visitors' feelings of being unwelcome. Familiarity with museums is often part of "a cultural code people acquire through their socialization in families and schools" (Bourdieu, quoted in Vom Lehn, Heath, & Hindmarsh, 2001, p. 192). More importantly, in the absence of access to personal connections in the galleries, visitors unfamiliar with museums may experience the space primarily as the site of numerous rules and unfamiliar structures (Dejkameh, Candiano, & Shipps, 2017, p. 10). The architectural features of a building may increase or impede accessibility to visitors with physical or intellectual disabilities. Additionally, a museum exhibition offering only visually presented works, accompanied only by written text, fails to provide sensory access to a wide range of visitors (Argyropoulos & Kanari, 2015).

Such restrictions of the aesthetic experience of museums can be productively expanded both through exhibitions and through educational and therapeutic interventions. In the realm of physical space, museums increasingly utilize physical contact in their galleries. The Victoria and Albert Museum in London displays "touch objects" in its galleries to increase the accessibility of artworks, understanding of materials, and understanding of technique (Hoskin, 2014). In New York, the Cooper Hewitt displayed an array of multisensory technologies used for understanding and enhancement in their 2018 exhibition *The Senses: Design Beyond Vision* (Cooper Hewitt, 2018). The long-running Art*Access* program at the Queens Museum, staffed by art therapists, was initiated in the early 1980s, with workshops using sculptural touch objects (Reyhani Dejkameh & Shipps, 2019).

As these touch object workshops have demonstrated, use of objects and programs may complement each other. Moreover, museum accessibility and relevance may be increased through programs. Both art educators and art therapists, sometimes in collaboration, have contributed to a broadened vision of the role of museums within society. Art therapists have expanded their practice into museums as uniquely appropriate settings (Coles, Harrison, & Todd, 2019; Peacock, 2012; Ioannides, 2016). Museum educators found that art therapists' educational and relational practices of art teaching have "therapeutic goals and outcomes" (Allison, 2013, p. 87), and that encounters with museum objects have inspired reminiscences, personal connection, and positive changes in mood during museum outreach programs (Chatterjee, Vreeland, & Noble, 2009; Smiraglia, 2015). The increased acceptance of museums as sites for art therapy reaffirms that "a community-based art therapy practice is a platform from which multiple narratives and exchanges can result in social change and individual empowerment" (Reyhani Dejkameh & Shipps, 2019, p. 211). Museum teaching is also enriched by "exploring the potential of the art museum as an environment that supports reflection, invites personal connections, and builds community" (Williams, 2010, p. 94).

Programs and groups in general can be understood as symbolic containing forms within the museum, and can both grow from and influence the mission and goals of a museum. Similar expressions of a museum's meaning, and primary access points for visitors who do not come into contact with programming opportunities are found in museum spaces and social texture, modes of communication, and interpretive materials. Some spatial influences are intentionally designed, while other interactions take place through the more fluid and unpredictable encounters between visitors and staff. A sense of interest and self-guided curiosity can stem from a feeling of agency during both programs and unstructured visits – at times, people resist implicit suggestions or alter their role in the expected performance of museums.

> Visitors slip through, leave a tour, swerve around an artist talk preferring to stroll slowly, engage in conversations, gaze at their cellular phone, go through different rhythms of slowness and speed while looking at the artworks and wandering through the gallery, or rest on a bench to read and quietly watch other visitors.
>
> (Berard, 2018, p. 96)

In galleries, options for exploring choice and interest are increased by use of multiple means of artistic presentation, interpretation, and engagement. Opportunities for moments of agency and glancing interaction with others are expanded for those who enter into museum artmaking spaces.

Exploring the Art Laboratory

Increasingly, art museums include a hands-on art room adjacent to the galleries. At the Museum of Modern Art in New York, for example, the Family Art Lab has occupied part of the adjacent Education Building for over a decade. When the redesigned museum opened in late 2019, it incorporated the additional Paula and James Crown Creativity Lab within the second floor of the main building, designed to host rotating interactive projects (Museum of Modern Art, 2019). MoMA has clearly prioritized adding experimental lab space closer to the galleries. Other museums nationwide, such as the Berkeley Art Museum and Pacific Film Archive and the Queens Museum (Lawrence, 2015; Queens Museum, 2019), have also expanded or developed similar spaces in recent years.

At the Museum of Craft and Design (MCD), developing the MakeArt Lab hands-on space was a process involving both the public programming priorities of staff and the physical qualities of the museum. The case study below explores the iterations of exhibition-specific artmaking piloted during 2019–20, but interest in and capacity for the drop-in space grew over previous years. Sarah Charlotte Jones, education director, brought her interest in developing a drop-in artmaking space to MCD when she began work in 2015, designing temporary in-gallery prototypes such as a "craft cart" to accompany particular exhibitions (Jones, personal communication, May 5, 2020). MCD held existing public programs on select days both in the galleries and MakeArt Lab space, including a Free First Tuesday program with an artmaking component. These programs, as well as interactive exhibitions during this time, received positive feedback from visitors. As a result, "there began to be more of an institutional alignment with ideas for making hands-on creativity accessible on a more consistent basis" (Jones, personal communication, May 5, 2020).

MCD, a non-collecting institution, was founded in 2004 and moved to its current San Francisco location in 2013. The museum's current layout is a relatively narrow rectangular floor plan occupying part of a larger building, with 4,000 square feet available for exhibitions (Museum of Craft and Design, 2013). Within that space, walls and dimensions are redesigned and changed with each exhibition. These range from a single show filling the space to as many as three exhibitions curated separately. After entering the building, passing the gift shop, and stepping into the ticketed museum proper, visitors would encounter a rectangular room perpendicular to the gallery space, dominated by a long metal table surrounded by chairs. Visitors could choose to participate in hands-on artmaking at any point when the room was publicly available and not in use as a staff meeting space. The gallery space could be seen directly outside the glass doors of the MakeArt Lab. Notably, "the glass doors were installed [in 2018] as an invitation to the space and to create more of a dynamic energy in the museum" (Jones, personal communication, May 5, 2020).

MCD prioritizes "making creativity accessible to everyone" (Museum of Craft and Design, 2019), and museum instruction and programming center on material and technique. The implied commitment of the room to providing an alternative means of accessing technique, concept, and material used in particular artists' works present a visual symbol of the museum's priorities and provide an additional level of accessibility. The identity of an institution is constructed by elements including its collection, style of textual interpretation, educational or therapeutic work with various publics, its online presence, and more. It may also be constructed with a characteristic interpretive perspective. Because MCD does not have a permanent collection, the display of its interpretive priorities comprises a large element of its public presentation.

Most hands-on projects at the MCD have traditionally involved an educator presenting one or more thematic or material elements in artworks featured in exhibitions and providing a prompt that inspires the creation of a completed, take-home project. The MakeArt Lab's open projects were conceptualized by Jones "as an additional interpretation tool for deeper exploration of the themes, materials, and techniques found in the exhibitions; an opportunity for visitors to rest and reflect; a social moment for intergenerational art-making amongst both families and strangers," with the hope that, for the public, "the opportunity to actually interact with contemporary craft and design processes and techniques will not just introduce them to the work and concepts, but will actually *involve* them" (Jones, personal communication, May 5, 2020). As outlined above, these efforts also addressed the accessibility of concepts: "not everyone learns and retains information in the same way, and traditional gallery/artwork/label methods of display can sometimes alienate certain learners" (Jones, personal communication, 2020).

Projects and Materials

In 2019–20, three cycles of projects took place, alongside particular exhibitions. The first iteration of projects in the open artmaking space was based on two artworks in the 2019 exhibition Material Domestication, curated by Elizabeth Kozlowski. Adam Shiverdecker's contribution to that group show was a monumental, multipiece work called *Banquet of Plutus*, a tableau hanging in space. Large wire armatures extended out of and completed the shape of numerous smooth, white, wheel-thrown Grecian-style vases and urns. Dark, scattered thin skins of clay also clung to a larger, centrally hanging armature with a vertical tail, evoking both a whale and a battered jet. To make the idea and function of an armature in Shiverdecker's work more tangible, and using a material in common with the artwork, Jones planned to use chicken wire as a base for clay additions. With some experimentation, a small, triangular, three-dimensional form took shape: small enough to sit on the table and somewhat roughly shaped, with all sharp edges protected, it functioned as a central but nondirectional focal point for visitors. Jones's initial plan for hands-on artmaking was a collaborative process following an aspect of Shiverdecker's approach: after flattening small balls of modeling clay, visitors were invited to gradually cover the structure, focusing as the artist had on shaping and playing with the exterior form.

Alongside the artwork inspired by Shiverdecker, the rest of the table was devoted to materials for a prompt based on the work of Jamie Bardsley, called *Palm Prints* (2019). Bardsley's original piece, directly outside of the MakeArt Lab, was composed of small, unglazed porcelain loops, each formed by the artist's hands and varying in size. Numerous visitors asked whether the balanced loops were made of paper or leather owing to their soft, matte surfaces. The porcelain shapes arrived at the museum as modular components stored according to size and were individually placed by Bardsley on the museum floor without adhesive, together forming a circle shape that rose and fell in height, not unlike a watery surface. In the MakeArt Lab, the work was referenced by a prompt to use small, repetitive shapes or marks to form a larger composition. Various pages of cardstock, lead and white pencils, and thin, fine-tipped markers were laid out as materials.

The second iteration of hands-on projects, organized over subsequent months in 2019, stemmed from the exhibition Dead Nuts: A Search for the Ultimate Machined Object. In this session, all three tables of the MakeArt Lab were given over to crafts based in metal and hardware materials, using the machined object as a starting point for creative explorations. At least four crafts were present at all times, and prompts varied between potentially wearable, functional projects, such as hex-nut or metal washer-woven jewelry, and more abstract explorations, such as hose clamps used as a frame and base for string, pipe cleaners, coated wire, and small hardware materials. Throughout the 4 months of this exhibition, a chess set composed of hardware materials was also available for use in the MakeArt Lab.

Finally, over the early weeks of 2020, hands-on activities were developed and publicly available relating to the work of exhibiting artist Linda Gass, whose work primarily consists of dyed silk tapestries depicting the effects of human activity on water sources and supply. Jones partnered with a local manufacturer of silk dye materials to secure paper-backed crepe-de-chine, acrylic dye, and resist. With these supplies, visitors were prompted to trace maps onto the silk surface, add resist lines, and dot in dye to fill the silk surface with various colors

Material Observations

In the first iteration of the MakeArt Lab's open space, the material choice of either adding clay to an armature or using pencils and marker to create repetitive patterns was significant. Pencils on paper are familiar, an association likely to create a feeling of control and familiarity within visitors (Regev & Snir, 2013). Paper and pencils were also placed at the side of the table closest to the door. Farther from the door, the triangular armature was centered on the table, with modeling clay balls prepared for visitors to manipulate and add on. Clay, in contrast to two-dimensional mark-making, can be manipulated, touched, and shaped in three dimensions, and even a slight touch effects a tangible change to the material (Sholt & Gavron, 2006, p. 68). The option to fully shape, observe, and transform clay was connected to the artist's work by the miniature armature. Pencils and markers on paper provided a symbolic link to Bardsley's artwork in its themes of repetition, abstraction, and cohesion of a larger artwork, but provided less of a direct material parallel.

As the first foray into open artmaking during museum hours, MCD's education staff expected that the paper, markers, and pencils provided might also serve as a surface for writing, drawing, and expressing reactions to the gallery spaces. This was sometimes the case. Many visitors did not follow the prompt to create clusters of marking within larger spaces. Some used pre-made sheets of abstract shapes to do so. Large drawings of people, symbols, and objects often emerged, though patterns also spread across many pages. Although museum signage invited visitors to bring their work with them, many participants left their artwork behind. MCD staff collected and saved all artworks on paper that remained.

Many visitors also did not follow the modeling clay station's written prompt to flatten the circles and place them against the armature, in a recollection of Shiverdecker's skin-like clay surfaces. A vast majority of the clay pieces left were easily identifiable as figurative: of animals, plants, people, and shapes. As the triangular chicken-wire armature had a flat top supported by vertical sides,

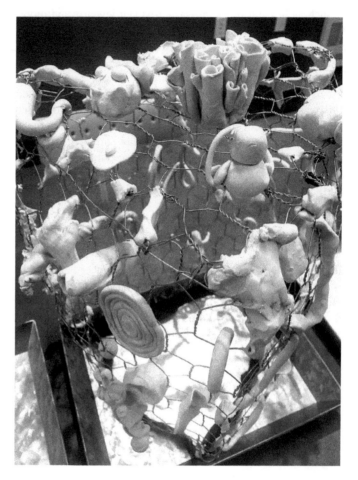

Figure 9.1 One expression of the collaborative armature project

visitors often chose to place their clay creations on top, with some layered on top of others' pieces. The orientation of the clay forms was not generally abstract or multidirectional, but was all the more exciting for its variety and the care expressed by participants in sculpting detail into such small figures (Figure 9.1).

Metal, as used in the MakeArt Lab projects that accompanied Dead Nuts, is a less familiar art material. For many educators and visitors, the idea of working with hardware material was new. The setup of the room, named "The Machinist Bar" during this time, also differed in the number of projects available. Typically, four projects were distributed across the table at any time: A type of wearable jewelry, one abstract project alternating between hose clamps and metal washer "weaving," an area with several large magnets on which visitors could build temporary towers using smaller hardware materials, and a hardware chess set built by the local Center Hardware. Two small "toddler tinker boards" were created by Jones to accompany the projects; these were oval wooden bases with larger hardware materials such as small wheels, locks, doorstops, and ties securely affixed. These proved popular. Young children and their caregivers were engaged by the tinker boards, and they attracted children and adults of other ages. The chess set and magnetic setup, though directly available to only two or three people at a given time, were also consistently popular with and intuitive to visitors. The chess set did not require conversation but invited sustained engagement in pairs and provided a different inroad to considering machined metal objects for visitors with different learning styles and skill levels. Familiar materials such as pipe cleaners and thread, which were intended for use with particular projects, were often successfully used on their own as more approachable introductions into the hands-on art-making process and were accessible to visitors with varied motor skills. Similarly, these softer materials, such as pipe cleaners, ribbon, and thread, provided a welcome connective counterpart to the solid metal objects. When educators were present in the MakeArt Lab, they observed the entry of visitors who were familiar with machined objects and parts, and these individuals were typically pleased to see the Art Lab setup despite its nontechnical nature. The chess set was a particular focus of such visitors.

One relevant feature of the room used for the MakeArt Lab was that its permanent walls do not have a solid ceiling. Sound from meetings, classes, conversations, and artmaking was audible outside in the nearby galleries and sometimes up to the front entry desk. The sound of washers and hex nuts on the metal table surface, and particularly that of metal pieces disconnecting from the large magnets, occasionally clattered through the gallery. These intermittent changes in the usually quiet atmosphere of the museum marked an exciting interruption by visitors into the overall impression of the museum, though it also may have potentially startled or unnerved other visitors.

In the concluding iteration of hands-on projects in early 2020, Dye-Na-Flow fabric dye was used on squares of silk after barriers had been created between colors with resist lines or shapes. This technique closely paralleled the process of exhibiting artist Linda Gass. Gass also uses thin lines of resist to separate dye colors and represent landforms on silk. Very few visitors to the MakeArt Lab were familiar with the properties of resist, of silk dye, or the process in general. Educators carefully introduced the project using straightforward textual instruction throughout the table and considered distribution of materials (e.g., small amounts of dye and single brushes made available in individual containers). Sharpie markers, which made more controlled dots and lines, were also provided. At times, when staff were present and able to observe the MakeArt Lab, they noted that visitors often appeared initially overwhelmed by the materials, but ultimately enjoyed the process. During this third iteration of the MakeArt Lab, long test strips of silk were taped across the entire center of the table, with existing spots of dye, and the table itself was covered in black paper. Jones tested and reordered the instructions so that prompts were included in close proximity to organized materials laid out on the table (i.e., resist, dye, pencils), as well as samples created by staff demonstrating different stages of the process.

One of the notable aspects of this most recent project was the required ongoing maintenance and cleanup. Throughout previous iterations of the publicly available MakeArt Lab projects, gallery guides and education staff replaced materials in containers, cleaned up papers, and replaced modeling clay, but, with the silk dyeing project, materials were more frequently moved from their point of origin. Numerous projects (still in the drying process) were left on the table, dyes were moved from their centralized tray, and small bottles of resist and silk squares were spread across the table. This project also required more frequent replacement of materials: the silk squares and paper-backed crepe-de-chine were cut from a much larger roll, and dyes needed regular replacement as well. However, the small dye bottles were not spilled, and colors were only very rarely mixed; mess and disarray were ultimately contained on the table.

Communication and Accessibility of the Museum and MakeArt Lab

MCD general admission cost $8 per person (in 2020), with free admission for children under 12, school groups, EBT/WiC holders, and NARM members, as well those who have received free passes during offsite public programs. During monthly Free First Tuesdays, a larger number of people were recorded visiting the MakeArt Lab than on a typical day. Staff made daily, varied efforts to alert visitors to the presence of the MakeArt Lab, including verbal notification, signage (including a sign hung on the door during staff meetings with the meeting's expected end time), and opening the doors when the room was free. Though art projects and informational signs in the MakeArt Lab were visible on the table from the galleries, passing through the glass doors still often required negotiation and questioning by visitors. While much consideration has been given to visually presented instruction in the space, additional auditory, Braille, or spoken staff interventions to bridge the gap for visitors who are blind or have low vision would have allowed more direct and wider access to the materials.

Because of the museum's relatively small size and its regularly changing layout and floor plan, the MakeArt Lab represented a more permanent physical feature of the institution. As drop-in, hands-on artmaking is the primary mode of public programming that takes place as part of MCD's regularly occurring programs, the content of the MakeArt Lab also informed visitors' understanding of the museum's goals and priorities. The museum always produces informational feedback regarding the architectural space, curatorial selections, and visitors, but the public MakeArt Lab added potential for more exchange – both implicit, between educators and visitors, and explicit, between staff and visitors engaged in the same room.

This pilot space provided a subjective, educator-designed intervention into the museum space, with a focus that changed completely with new exhibitions. Making no attempt to address each and every work of art or artist on view, the lab made visible a bit of "of the unconscious mental life of the institution and its activities of curating, collecting, conserving and educating" (Froggett & Trustram, 2014, p. 484). An ethos of educational and creative choice was modeled by this approach, making interpretive processes visible and modeling such choices for visitors. The presence of hands-on elements gave wider audiences access to different ways of engaging with the exhibit, as people with varied learning styles and abilities were invited to engage in processes of exploration.

The underlying message of these interpretive choices is that meaning may extend in many directions. A project prompt such as the metal-focused Machinist Bar is particularly representative: many different project interpretations developed from a single material, for many different ages and developmental stages across the life span, were represented. As "good teaching is not simply a matter of transmitting knowledge but is rather an experience that stimulates knowledge construction" (Moon, 2012, p. 193), even these types of implicit teaching can carry forward examination and experimentation with the material and technical aspects of an exhibition, producing potential learning and knowledge. Along these lines, Jones also hopes that such hands-on projects "will not just introduce [visitors] to the work and concepts, but will actually *involve* them – resulting in the coveted outcome of having visitors connect with the subject matter by actually seeing themselves reflected in the galleries" (Jones, personal correspondence, May 5, 2020). Ideally, in a creative exchange that "blurs the boundaries between 'production' and 'consumption' involving both sides in the making of pluralized meanings, perspectives and subjectivities" (Schorch, 2013, p. 204), visitors have a way to communicate their own interpretations of artworks to the museum outside of the provided prompts. Indeed, visitors sometimes communicated these reinterpretations through their artwork, by expanding the subjects of the prompts in new directions: using drawing paper to document experience or reflection, meticulously sculpting a clay figure, creating a fantastical, jellyfish-like sculpture out of metal and pipe cleaners, or using silk dye to form abstract shapes, diverging from the artist referents.

In this museum, and with this particular material way of relating to the exhibits, visitors choosing to engage in the activities of the MakeArt Lab would not necessarily "select cultural objects of personal significance and elaborate their relations to them" (Pantagoutsou, Ioannides, & Vaslamatzis, 2017, p. 75) as one might do in a group or tour when handling or viewing a culturally weighted or personally significant object. Yet the shared project brought them closer to the possibility of connection and shared communication, which would be enhanced even further with the steady presence of a facilitator. In my observations, participants frequently made art quietly in parallel with other small groups; sometimes new familial or group dynamics, such as a child leading activities or parent enjoying a lengthy sensory craft experience, were observed within the group (Silverman, 1989, p. 142). When observers and theorists have placed emphasis on even incidental contact between visitors as catalysts for how they may "come to experience an exhibit in highly contingent and situationally relevant ways" (Vom Lehn et al., 2001, p. 202), shared space and parallel purpose are significant. Even more importantly, "creating similar artworks in response to an object can further highlight shared feelings and experiences" (Coles et al., 2019, p. 61).

The MakeArt Lab underwent a process of iterative change as a drop-in space, and staff sought out visitor feedback to inform further updates and refinements. It is worthwhile to ask, in considering intellectual and conceptual understanding, "where such activity leads: whether it restricts the meaning of the artwork to its formal similarities to other artworks, as Bourdieu suggests, or leads *through* the artwork to spaces of the imagination" (Nespor, 2000, p. 22). However, the MakeArt Lab concept and space are still in the process of experimentation and change. There may well be more conceptual ties and embodied inroads to deeper layers of tactile, auditory, or personal and historical contexts for the artists, which would deepen imaginative connections and lead to new understanding. Meanwhile, information theorists and researchers alike have found that "sensory engagements . . . open the gates to imagination as an integral dimension of any meaning" (Schorch, 2013, p. 205). There is a continuity, as discussed above, with exhibitions of centuries ago, in which "a hands-on approach to exhibits enabled visitors to acquire an embodied understanding of the nature of the display" (Classen, 2007, p. 901). Given that visitors of all abilities seek out and enjoy "exact replicas of the originals so they can be actively touched, tactual models and tactile diagrams" (Argyropoulos & Kanari, 2015, p. 138), the MakeArt Lab provided an excellent setting for comfortably exploring such tactile models, as well as additional reading or audio materials, in multiple formats, and opportunities for visitors to sit at length and explore exhibition publications. As the room's title of 'Lab' signaled a commitment to exploration and experimentation, further possibilities were readily suggested, and could be well developed in conjunction with visitors and other museum partners.

A final element of educational transparency is present in a challenging feature of the MakeArt Lab: as noted above, it was not available to visitors at all times. The challenge of this situation could arise when repeat visitors become used to their relationship with the museum being informed and interpreted through hands-on interactives and yet are not able to rely on the room's openness on a given day. However, the inner workings of the museum were uniquely visible in this setting, conveying an impression of openness and imparting some understanding of the museum's own cultural context to visitors. If knowledge of the roles of museum workers gives context to the museum's meaning and increased understanding of participation to visitors (Garoian, 2001, p. 247), there is some value in the openness and unexpectedness of such information. Similarly, the necessity of staff checking up on the lab and providing visible signs of care to the space added to a feeling of connection to the visitor – necessary for the staff as much as for participants – and visibility.

However, this examination must note that the third iteration of the MakeArt Lab's participatory pilot space closed several months ahead of schedule owing to the spread of the COVID-19 virus across the country, with potential lasting effects on museums. With the closure of physical spaces, many universities, museums, and other points of public contact have provided newly accessible digital resources, often those long sought by activists and educators (Hamraie, 2020). The cultural holding spaces of museums have shifted their form. With fewer people traveling between spaces, and such vigorous online production, this is a good time for reflection on the ways that typical social, physical, and cultural expectations and paradigms shape societal perceptions of who is able, interested, and part of a desired audience. MCD initiated and shared new digital craft instructions on its website in the first weeks of California's shelter guidelines, bringing a longtime goal into immediate usage, and staff characteristically began thinking about ways the museum could be involved outside its walls. However, back in the museum, reopening will also necessarily include safety procedures that restrict the sharing of materials (CIMAM, 2020), erode some of the pleasure of sharing the experience of cultural spaces, restrict numbers of visitors and their proximity, and likely bring a heightened sense of trepidation and watchfulness into the experience of museums. In the wake of fear surrounding the sharing of objects and the proximity of others, museums may choose to employ the interpretive skills of staff to rely more on verbal and written communications with visitors in the gallery spaces, while hands-on activities may temporarily be replaced by objects designated for single use by individuals only or may undergo frequent cleaning. With trust and communication as the valuable core of making galleries welcoming, staff will need to use their skills of extending welcome and a message of accessibility in new ways, and museums as a whole will require awareness of changes in their specific series of cultural holding containers. The flexibility, commitment to access, reciprocal exchange with audiences, and attention to personal connection demonstrated in many online museum communications will be needed in the galleries and artmaking spaces.

References

Allison, A. (2013). Old friends, bookends: Art educators and art therapists. *Art Therapy*, *30*(2), 86–89. doi:10.1080/07421656.2013.787215

Argyropoulos, V. S., & Kanari, C. (2015). Reimagining the museum through "touch": Reflections of individuals with visual disabilities on their experience of museum-visiting in Greece. *ALTER, European Journal of Disability Research, 9*, 130–143.

Berard, M.-F. (2018). Strolling along with Walter Benjamin's concept of the flâneur and thinking of art encounters in the museum. In A. L. Cutcher & R. L. Irwin (Eds.), *The flâneur and education research: A metaphor for knowing, being ethical and new data production* (93–108). Cham, Switzerland: Springer International.

Chatterjee, H., Vreeland, S., & Noble, G. (2009). Museopathy: Exploring the healing potential of handling museum objects. *Museum and Society, 7*(3), 164–177.

CIMAM. (2020, April 29). Precautions for museums during covid-19 pandemic. https://cimam.org/resources-publications/precautions-museums-during-covid-19-pandemic/

Classen, C. (2007). Museum manners: The sensory life of the early museum. *Journal of Social History, 40*(4), 895–914.

Coles, A., Harrison, F., & Todd, S. (2019). Flexing the frame: Therapist experiences of museum-based group art psychotherapy for adults with complex mental health difficulties. *International Journal of Art Therapy, 24*(2), 56–67.

Cooper Hewitt. (2018). The senses: Design beyond vision. www.cooperhewitt.org/channel/senses/

Dejkameh, M. R., Candiano, J., & Shipps, R. (2017). Paving new ways to exploration in cultural institutions: A gallery guide for inclusive arts-based engagement in cultural institutions. Queensmuseum.org. www.queensmuseum.org/wp-content/uploads/2018/02/PAVE%20Guide_web.pdf

Froggett, L. & Trustram, M. (2014). Object relations in the museum: A psychosocial perspective. *Museum Management and Curatorship, 29*(5), 482–497.

Garoian, C. R. (2001). Performing the museum. *Studies in Art Education, 42*(3), 234–248.

Hamraie, A. (2020, March 10). Accessible teaching in the time of Covid-19. Mapping access. www.mapping-access.com/blog-1/2020/3/10/accessible-teaching-in-the-time-of-covid-19

Hoskin, D. (2014, June 4). Please touch. V&A blog. www.vam.ac.uk/blog/creating-new-europe-1600-1800-galleries/please-touch

Hubard, O. M. (2007). Complete engagement: Embodied response in art museum education. *Art Education, 60*(6), 46–56.

Ioannides, E. (2016). Museums as therapeutic environments and the contribution of art therapy. *Museum International, 68*(3–4), 98–109. doi:10.1111/muse.12125

Lawrence, A. (2015). Diller Scofidio + Renfro unveils its design for the Berkeley Art Museum and Pacific Film Archive. *Architectural Digest*. Retrieved June 2, 2020, from: www.architecturaldigest.com/story/bam-pfa-diller-scofidio-and-renfro-new-building

Moon, B. L. (2012). Art therapy teaching as performance art. *Art Therapy: Journal of the American Art Therapy Association, 29*(4), 192–195.

Museum of Craft and Design. (2013, April). Welcome to Dogpatch. https://sfmcd.org/welcome-to-dogpatch/

Museum of Craft and Design. (2019, December). About the museum. https://sfmcd.org/aboutmcd/

Museum of Modern Art. (2019, October). The people's studio. www.moma.org/calendar/groups/7

Nespor, J. (2000). School field trips and the curriculum of public spaces. *Journal of Curriculum Studies, 32*(1), 25–43.

Palmer, A. (2008). Untouchable: Creating desire and knowledge in museum costume and textile exhibitions. *Fashion Theory, 12*(1), 31–63.

Pantagoutsou, A., Ioannides, E., & Vaslamatzis, G. (2017). Exploring the museum's images – Exploring my image (Exploration des images du musée, exploration de mon image), *Canadian Art Therapy Association Journal, 30*(2), 69–77

Peacock, K. (2012). Museum education and art therapy: Exploring an innovative partnership. *Art Therapy: Journal of the American Art Therapy Association, 29*(3), 133–137.

Queens Museum. (2019). Queens Museum launches Cities of Tomorrow Art Lab. https://queensmuseum.org/2019/04/cities-of-tomorrow-art-lab

Regev, D. & Snir, S. (2013). Art therapy for treating children with autism spectrum disorders (ASD): The unique contribution of art materials. *The Academic Journal of Creative Arts Therapies, 3*(2), 251–260.

Reyhani Dejkameh, M., & Shipps, R. (2019). From please touch to Art*Access*: The expansion of a museum-based art therapy program. *Art Therapy: Journal of the American Art Therapy Association, 35*(4), 211–217.

Schorch, P. (2013). The experience of a museum space. *Museum Management and Curatorship. 28*(2). doi:10.1080/09647775.2013.776797

Sholt, M., & Gavron, T. (2006). Therapeutic qualities of clay-work in art therapy and psychotherapy: A review. *Art Therapy: Journal of the American Art Therapy Association, 23*(2), 66–72.

Silverman, L. (1989). Johnny showed us the butterflies. *Marriage & Family Review, 13*(3–4), 131–150.

Smiraglia, C. (2015). Museum programming and mood: Participant responses to an object-based reminiscence outreach program in retirement communities. *Arts & Health, 7*(3), 187–201.

Vom Lehn, D., Heath, C., & and Hindmarsh, J. (2001). Exhibiting interaction: Conduct and collaboration in museums and galleries. *Symbolic Interaction, 24*(3), 189–216.

Williams, R. (2010). Honoring the personal response: A strategy for serving the public hunger for connection. *The Journal of Museum Education, 35*(1), 93–102.

10 There's Always Room at the Table

The Art Hive of the Montreal Museum of Fine Arts

Stephen Legari

At the stroke of 3 pm, regular participants are already through the door and securing their favorite spots. Some prefer to be close to the many shelves of materials, others like to be near the towering plants, while another takes advantage of the still quiet room by stretching out their art project on a long wooden table. Paint is poured out, magazines are scoured through, ongoing projects are retrieved and revived, and the din of creative activity begins to fill the space. In the next 5 hours, there may be anywhere between 15 and 50 people who either happen across the Art Hive of the Montreal Museum of Fine Arts (MMFA) or have made it their destination. Diverse in their reasons for accessing a community studio embedded in a fine art museum, they manage to find and create common ground. On the best days, generations, abilities, genders, languages, ethnicities, and materials co-mingle in an unprogrammed harmony – and sometimes playful cacophony.

The MMFA inaugurated its Art Hive in April of 2017. The community studio was established on the successful dissemination of the art hive model (arthives.org), which has seen dozens of hives spring up across the city of Montreal in recent years, and more than 200 across the world. The Art Hive at the MMFA is a university–museum partnership with Concordia University that sees the studio at the intersection of the diverse museum practices of the Division of Education and Wellness (DEW) that include art therapy, well-being, social inclusion, community outreach, diversity, and healthcare research partnerships. The evolution of these practices is well documented elsewhere (Legari, Lajeunesse, & Giroux, 2020); therefore, this discussion will confine its focus to the Art Hive.

In this chapter, the Art Hive is presented as both a literal space and a theoretical framework for the implementation of participatory spaces in museums that seek to empower members of the public not only as recipients of culture, but as actors in its shaping. In the following pages, the theory and practice that inform an art hive within a fine art museum context will be explored, relevant literature cited, the relationship to community art therapy studios established, and excerpts from long-time participants quoted to assist in bringing the studio to life within these pages.

DOI: 10.4324/9781003014386–10

Community Art Therapy Studios: Theory and Practice

The Art Hive community studio model, now more than 20 years in developed applied practice (Timm-Bottos, 1995), weaves together a number of histories in art therapy, community organizing, civil rights, crafter collectives, and social justice and grounds the international network in common values and practice. According to the Art Hive Network,

> The Art Hive Network connects small and regenerative community arts studios together in order to build solidarity across geographic distances. This effort seeks to strengthen and promote the benefits of these inclusive, welcoming spaces across Canada, and throughout the world. Also known as "public homeplaces," these third spaces create multiple opportunities for dialogue, skill sharing, and art making between people of differing socio-economic backgrounds, ages, cultures and abilities.
>
> (Arthives, n.d.)

For the purposes of this discussion, the connection of the art hives to art therapy and museum-based art therapy will be explored, given that the Art Hive of the MMFA is affiliated with a museum art therapy program and the Creative Arts Therapies Department of Concordia University. The reader is encouraged to explore the literature on art hives and the network website for a broader and more in-depth history of the model and its various applications (Timm-Bottos, 1995, 2006, 2011, 2016, 2017; Timm-Bottos & Reilly, 2014).

The open studio, community art therapy, the community art therapy studio, and the Art Hive all share important characteristics, but also distinctions. For art therapists, these distinctions inform the parameters of practice and proximity to clinical or clinically informed work.

Open studio art therapy has a long and diverse history dating back to those studios found in psychiatric and rehabilitation institutions during the years following World War II (Adamson & Timlin, 1984; Malchiodi, 2007). Open studio art therapy does not have one determined set of prescribed practices, but generally encompasses several ethically sound principles in common that differentiate it from closed-group or individual clinical art therapy. These principles include the opportunity for art therapists to make work alongside their clients; the normalizing of the display of artworks in the space, which has shown to be beneficial (Matton & Plante, 2014); the empowerment of the group to make choices about materials, pacing, and objectives; a de-emphasizing of pathology; and often flexibility around time and attendance (Hyland Moon, 2016). In Quebec, the art therapy open studio has been an active practice for decades, with several devoted, across the province, to different populations, predominantly those dealing with mental health issues (Sokoloff, 2019).

Community art therapy shares many of the same principles as the open studio but trains its energy on community empowerment. Ottemiller and Awais

(2016) propose a model of community art therapy that works from a "holistic, wellness, and strengths-based perspective" (p. 148) and supports the community's efforts to co-support each other, effecting change on a systemic level, which may in turn benefit the individual. This approach emphasizes the community as creative collaborators and community empowerment and, rather than a group of individual clients, sees the community as the client with collectively motivated goals and strengths to achieve them (Kapitan, Litell, & Torres, 2011; Ottemiller & Awais, 2016)

The development of community art therapy benefits from the art therapist stretching their skill set beyond the clinic and the hospital to bring vital diversity and inclusiveness to an ever-developing range of art therapy practice (Ottemiller & Awais, 2016). This approach champions flexibility and an anti-oppressive stance by working outside of the medical model. As Nolan (2019) writes,

> art therapists who practice in a community setting address client-generated goals without the constraints of mental health treatment . . . [and] . . . strive to foster in participants a sense of personal and collective agency through expression and feelings of belonging and purpose while furthering healthy connections within the group.
>
> (pp. 77–78)

The community studio approach, often associated with the work of Pat Allen (Allen, 1995), initially took a step further away from notions or practices of therapy or art therapy where the art therapist divested themselves of their therapeutic title. The art therapist would embed themselves as an artmaker within the community, while keeping an eye to holding space compassionately but at more of a distance than that of a therapist. This approach would go on to influence a range of community studio practices that maintain various degrees of connection to their clinical art therapy roots. As Allen (2008) writes,

> Rather than focusing on the therapeutic relationship, the open studio process seeks to promote the relationship between each of us and the artist within, or the self with the soul . . . The community studio, as we conceive it, is a place of all possibility, where anything can be expressed as a moment on life's continuum . . . Community studios vary in terms of which customs and procedures of a mental health program they retain, if any.
>
> (p. 11)

Somewhere in the cross-pollination of the open studio, community art therapy, and the community studio is the community art therapy studio. Community art therapy studios form an approach that benefits from these different linages of practice, both within different art therapy disciplines (e.g., community and clinical art therapy) and without, such as practices in arts-based community organizing. While there are transferable skills between the clinical and community domains of art therapy, and indeed between facilitating closed groups, open studios, and community studios, community art therapy studios are an approach unto their own. The community art therapy studio is a co-created space both in theory and practice (Nolan, 2019). The triangular relationship traditionally facilitated between client, art, and art therapist is extended to the community studio and, hence, the community. In her research, Nolan (2019) noted an absence of identified means of transformation in the community art therapy studio. In her narrative synthesis on the experiences of art therapists working through a community studio framework, Nolan (2019) identifies three salient themes that inform the mechanism of change in the studio participant: they are "safety, acceptance, and opportunity within healthy relationships" (p. 78).

Seen along the aforementioned continuum of studio art therapy practice, the Art Hive is perhaps the most diffuse in its resemblance to classic open studio art therapy, but finds common ground in both community art therapy and community studio practice.

The MMFA Art Hive in Practice

With a mandate of arts-based social inclusion, the Art Hive of the MMFA opens its doors twice a week to the public at large and provides free access to materials, space, time, and the expertise of facilitators for sessions that can last up to 5 hours. The Art Hive at the MMFA is not, exclusively speaking, a community art therapy studio. Although it is always co-facilitated by one or more art therapists, it also benefits from the presence of one of the museum's mediators (the title applied at the MMFA to those professionals who have a specialization in art education and art history). It is perhaps more accurate to conceive of the Art Hive as informed by community art therapy studio practice. But, given its position within a fine art museum, it is perhaps a sub-model unto itself that finds some affiliation with other institutional art hives such as those found in universities.

Like Allen (2008), Timm-Bottos de-emphasizes the overt facilitating role of the art therapist and calls for a public practice that can include a variety of people in facilitating roles, including artists, social workers, art educators, volunteers, and participants from the community itself (Timm-Bottos, 2017). The art hives strive to blur the lines between facilitator and participant, between clinical and public practice, between pedagogy and lived experience, and between therapy and community wellness to benefit and welcome everyone, especially those living in the margins (Timm-Bottos, 2016). Those facilitating at the hive practice the radical hospitality espoused by the hive's founder, which finds congruence in the museum's humanistic stance (Bondil, 2016).

Upon arrival, each participant is greeted, welcomed, and oriented to the space and materials. From there, each is invited to develop autonomously, at their own pace. Searching the shelves laden with materials, including those ready to be upcycled, the artist-participant is encouraged to struggle through the choices and creative problem solving, which is believed to benefit both the individual and the community. The art therapist and the mediator remain on hand to support, listen, collaborate, and attend to the flow of the room. The work, when done well, can appear invisible but may call on all the resources of the facilitators, depending on the complexity of need of the individual and the community. The collaboration between facilitators and participants serves to disrupt hierarchy and instill a sense of co-created safety for which everyone is responsible. The quality of presence of the facilitators is an essential component of the art hive atmosphere and sense of a safe-enough space for any participant or family to find their place at the table. As Timm-Bottos (2006) writes, "the studio staff, including art therapists and regularly participating artists, establishes a base line of security within the creative community atmosphere, nonverbally inviting the visiting child or adult to continue his or her relational attachment works" (p. 18).

A Third Place in a Fine Art Museum

Third space (Bhaba, 2012) and third place (Elmborg, 2011) theory inform the practice at the art hives, including that at the MMFA (Timm-Bottos & Reilly, 2014). In practical terms, third places are those that encourage community but are neither a primary (home) or secondary (e.g., work) place, the availability of which is positively associated with a better quality of life (Jeffres et al., 2009). Third places exist in the figurative interstitial borderland of culture and the literal place that welcomes the participant into a collectively created environment of exchange and belonging. Third spaces seek to disrupt hierarchy, emphasize the multiplicity of lived experience, and empower those whose voices have traditionally been marginalized (Elmborg, 2011; Timm-Bottos, 2011). While third places can be gathering places of any and many kinds within a community, both libraries and museums have been conceived of as third places (Elmborg, 2011; Evans & Dubowski, 2001; Murzyn-Kupisz & Działek, 2015). As Rowson Love and Szymanski (2017) explain,

> A third place . . . is place a to rejuvenate and reflect, but more importantly it is about conversation and social action . . . It is inclusive, welcoming both regulars and newcomers . . . as systems thinking moves us toward more community embeddedness and social engagement, many museums seek to become more relevant as third spaces.
>
> (p. 196)

The notion of a participatory space in a museum is certainly not without precedent. Arts-based participatory projects have become integrated into many museum mandates alongside the more traditional education activities. But what the art hive manages to activate is a sustained presence of participatory energy that responds to Simon's (2010) call for de-hierarchization between facilitators and public. This notion is congruent with Timm-Bottos's emphasis on a more horizontal participation of the art hive facilitator, who may hold space but also learns, creates, and participates as a member of the community (Timm-Bottos, 2006). Upon entering the art hive, it is not uncommon to wonder who is a participant and who is a facilitator.

The Art Hive at the MMFA responds to a call for museums to embrace both systems thinking and third place/space practice (Rowson Love & Szymanski, 2017). The conception of the museum as a self-contained ecosystem is helpful for grasping its many moving and interconnected parts, and how an art hive both complements and intervenes within this ecosystem. As a community studio, the space and practice are unlike any other within the museum and yet have become entirely woven into the greater fabric of the museum institution.

If the lines are successfully blurred, then the hive helps the museum lean towards Simon's (2010) ambition for museums to achieve a stage of participatory development wherein "the entire institution feel[s] social, full of potentially interesting, challenging, enriching encounters with other people" (p. 27). In imagining the bidirectional influence of the Art Hive on the art museum and vice versa, Canas (2011, n.p.) posits:

> The encounter between an institution and its community may be of a quality that exceeds previous modes of interaction, so that the institution does not act as the institution but is rather willing to step outside its comfort role. Can the art museum solicit the help of its community in creating, interpreting, or promoting art? Can this wavering from the institutionalized role speak to a willingness to be changed, to be acculturated along with and beside its previously unacknowledged neighbours?

Research

Museum-based art therapy has progressively produced a variety of literature demonstrating the benefits for various publics and populations of art therapy offered in museum settings (Coles & Harrison, 2017; Coles & Jury, 2020; Ioannides, 2016; Sloan, 2013; Treadon, Rosal, & Thompson Wylder, 2006). To this, the MMFA has added its own contributions to research in this specialized practice of art therapy, including studies exploring the benefits of museum art therapy for people living with eating disorders, the history of art therapy in a fine art museum, and of art therapy supervision in a fine art museum (Baddeley et al., 2017; Henry, Parker, & Legari, 2019; Legari et al., 2020; Thaler et al., 2017). Community approaches to art therapy have also been explored through museums (Parashak, 1997; Rosenblatt, 2014; Stiles & Mermer-Welly, 1998). In this vein, in 2018, the MMFA hosted a mixed-methods pilot study that used an art hive-informed art therapy protocol and showed benefits in several domains for young adults living with epilepsy (Smallwood, Legari, & Sheldon, 2020).

Model

The Art Hive of the MMFA is proposed as a museum-based community art and art therapy studio model that may serve to influence how other museums conceive of and implement community spaces in their institutions. The benefits of such a model include (1.) an ongoing participatory space that encourages museum participants and visitors to reflect on and influence the environment around them; (2.) a non-programmed, facilitated, inclusive space that has a strengths-based focus; (3.) a dynamic hub where participants can encounter each other safely and creatively while feeling supported; (4.) a third place/ space that impacts both community culture and museum culture reciprocally; and (5.) a multifunctional environment that can serve as a community studio, a studio for closed groups, an aftercare destination for closed-group participants, and a space for teaching. The Art Hive at the MMFA opens, both literally and figuratively, a new door of entry into the museum where previously marginalized participants can find and create their own space.

The museum art hive can also be conceived within a larger ecosystem of the museum's ongoing activities and spaces. Guides, educators, exhibitions, curation, and points of entry may influence the participation at the hive and vice versa. A first-time exhibition visitor may find the door to the hive on their way to another gallery space. A guide may mention the presence of a community studio to a group. The flow of a visit through the permanent collection may be interrupted by the compelling sight of people creating. And the hive participant may likewise find themselves drawn to unknown parts of the museum based on recommendation or invitation. The interplay between the museum's collections and staff functions organically rather than deliberately. The unprogrammed exploration of materials may be recreated in the galleries through a spirit of wonder and wander.

The Art Hive of the MMFA is also an institutional model that can be adapted to other museums. At the time of writing, both the Musée des beaux-arts de Sherbrooke, in Sherbrooke, Quebec, and the Agnes Etherington Art Centre, located on the campus of Queens University in Kingston, Ontario, had integrated art hives into their programming.

The Bees

There are many different ways in which the participants of the Art Hive at the MMFA find their way to the studio. As a part of the Art Hive Network, many participants will explore different art hives, both near and far, and will refer others when they have found something they like. It is not uncommon for a new participant to have been referred by an existing one, and word of mouth remains the most often used method of communicating the existence of a hive and its offering. Given its location within a fine art museum, many participants happen upon the studio by chance during their visit to an exhibit or the galleries. Participants who have completed other activities, including closed art therapy groups, will be referred to the Art Hive as a kind of aftercare. And finally, participants may also be referred through official channels such as through a social worker, psychologist, creative arts therapist, or even through our museum prescription program, available to collaborating family doctors in Quebec. The following are testimonies from a sampling of those who have participated in and shaped the evolution of the Art Hive of the MMFA since its debut.

Stacey maintains a regular, twice-weekly presence at the hive. She is quick to jump in and welcome newcomers and believes strongly in the Art Hive's role and presence in the museum. She has often expressed a strong affinity for the museum, its collections, its spaces, and its publics. Stacey moves with curious hands from one form of artmaking to another and both contributes to and benefits from the social dimension of the studio.

> When I came here I was so broken; I had so many issues, and pain, and everything. And art at the Musée has allowed me to do the things that are most difficult for me, which is make friends, talk to people, network, to be truly accepted and open with other artists. That is the role of art at the Museum. The point is art as healer in a safe community. For the people that are not interested in therapy, that are looking to get well on their own, that are looking to fight off depression, physical pain, anguish, monotony, boredom and broken dreams, Musée des Beaux Arts is where it's at. You just walk her halls, and she just begs you to see beyond the humdrum. I started volunteering, I have a hope, a future and a dream for my life.
>
> (Stacey, regular hive participant and volunteer since 2017)

Gerry will dive into any conversation and is deft at exploring art history, world cultures, engineering, and mental health and is always quick to say something positive about the studio. He can be found at the Art Hive nearly every hour it is open. Now retired from more than one career, his work benefits from years of experience as a sculptor and sculpting technician, but his approach to material in the here and now is very much about play. While Gerry can tell you the intricacies of working with bronze, he seems to derive equal pleasure from working with melted plasticine. He never fails to alight when someone expresses interest in learning.

> Coming here gives me an opportunity to come back in time and sculpt again. I don't want to teach for money and I don't want to sell my art for money anymore; I want it to be an ongoing sense of pleasure. Money distorts your path; you can't really do what you want to do. At the time when I was doing sculpture, if you look at my work, it was about being noticed, it was about being grand and shocking. Gargoyles and distorted figures . . .

Now, at this time in my life, it doesn't matter what people think. I'm a volunteer here, if somebody wants to learn anything. I like teaching, because you get a sense of accomplishment when somebody else does things right. Even if they're better than you, it's great! It's detachment from your own ego, and a sense of gratification.

(Gerry, regular hive participant and volunteer since 2017)

Arriving from Martinique for an extended stay with her son in Montreal, Yveline took to the art hive as if it were an extension of her existing practice. She expertly manipulated all manner of up-cyclable materials into two- and three-dimensional works of art. Her mixed media work blended both the figurative and the abstract and expressed freedom and her encounters with other cultures.

I am a painter and visual artist, I come from Martinique. [In 2017] I decided to go out into the world. I was a teacher of applied art and I had finished my career, so I decided to refine my artistic work even more, and to discover in other countries what art is and what art can bring to a human being. Because I think that art is an activity that can enrich life in all aspects, in all the values that we are losing. I too did a training in art therapy, so I was delighted to know that here, we could have a structure to allow each individual, in all simplicity, to have a place where we can share all that we have as richness, and all that we have as faults as well.

(Yveline, regular hive participant since 2017)

Yan Yee Poon has been a facilitating art therapist with the MMFA Art Hive since its launch in 2017. Like many art therapists, her skills have been honed in a variety of settings, including clinical and community, with groups and individuals. At the hive she brings this wealth of experience to the service of the ever-evolving community studio. As was previously explored, the art therapist in the community studio does not leave aside the complexity of their training but rather adapts it to the moment-to-moment unfolding of the studio dynamic. In the Art Hive, the facilitators, be they art therapists or educators, are encouraged to make, share, and collaborate with and through artmaking. This modelling often appears as an extension of the warmth and care that begins in the greetings of participants. However, those facilitating are not immune to the benefits of the community studio approach.

As an art therapist, the creative and nurturing space of the Hive offered me a place to practice being comfortable with boundaries that fluctuate and challenged my habitual ways of seeing and being. The roles are not set in stone; each moment spent there is a dance. There is a continuous interweaving of roles, from learner to teacher, from storyteller to listener, from art maker to supporter; we all learn to practice this dance with open hearts. My work at the Hive also reminds me of the importance of self-care, to feed our souls with creative expression, not just as a witness but an active participant. It taught me about authenticity and vulnerability and that who I am as a person and what I bring is important and welcomed as well.

(Yan Yee Poon, art therapist)

Challenges and Discussion

The Art Hive of the MMFA has greeted an annual average of about 2000 participants. Tourists, visitors, regulars, artists, patients, families, and museum employees represent just some of the multiple profiles of those who come, whether out of curiosity to create, or to find community. There are basic logistical challenges in accommodating numbers, though somehow the team at the Art Hive always manages to find space for one more. The studio follows a drop-in format, allowing for a natural flow of those coming and going.

At the heart of the art hive model is a practice of arts-based social inclusion that seeks to welcome everyone and especially those who have been marginalized. Social isolation has been shown to negatively impact both physical and psychological health and is associated with poor quality of life (Leigh-Hunt et al., 2017). The Art Hive is a response to the grave problem of social isolation and proposes an antidote through community-driven creative activity and connection. The effects of social isolation, however, do not remain at the door, and it can be challenging to support participants whose needs are complex. Art therapists are well placed to support those who live with the effects of illness, trauma, and social isolation, and community studios benefit from their range of competencies including skills in active listening, validation, redirection through artmaking, and de-escalation. Likewise, the museum mediators who share the facilitation responsibilities at the Art Hive of the MMFA are well versed in working with a range of publics and are essential allies in supporting and maintaining the community. As Allen (2008) writes,

> All cultural workers – whether more closely aligned to health care or to the art world – have the capacity to increase our mutual recognition of one another as valued members of our respective societies. Art can hold and express all that it means to be human. We should embrace and aid in the proliferation of places – of all varieties – where the basic human right of artistic self-expression is cherished and enjoyed.
>
> (p. 12)

In May of 2020, the studio had both marked its third anniversary and been bereft of participants for nearly 2 months. At the time of writing, COVID-19 had forced the temporary closure of the Art Hive of the MMFA. Across the Art Hive Network, facilitators and volunteers have set up virtual, pop-up hives to fill the gap in connecting through creating while innovating new uses for technology using the hive model. Many participants, however, including some regulars from the MMFA Hive, remain without a reliable internet connection and are left waiting for the coast to be clear and the doors to open once again. COVID-19 will have an indelible impact on how we practice arts-based social inclusion in a museum setting, where physical distancing and safety will be a priority for an uncertain time to come.

References

Adamson, E., & Timlin, J. (1984). *Art as healing*. London: Nicolas-Hays.
Allen, P. B. (1995). Coyote comes in from the cold: The evolution of the open studio concept. *Art Therapy*, *12*(3), 161–166. https://doi.org/10.1080/07421656.1995.107 59153
Allen, P. B. (2008). Commentary on community-based art studios: Underlying principles. *Art Therapy*, *25*(1), 11–12. https://doi.org/10.1080/07421656.2008.10129350
Arthives. (n.d.). Art hives. Retrieved from www.arthives.org
Baddeley, G., Evans, L., Lajeunesse, M., & Legari, S. (2017). Body talk: Examining a collaborative multiple-visit program for visitors with eating disorders. *Journal of Museum Education*, *42*(4), 345–353. https://doi.org/10.1080/10598650.2017. 1379278
Bhaba, H. K. (2012). *The location of culture* (2nd ed.). London: Routledge.
Bondil, N. (2016). Manifesto for a humanist museum. In N. Bondil (Ed.), *Michal and Renata Hornstein: Pavilion for peace* (124). Montreal: Montreal Museum of Fine Arts.
Canas, E. (2011). Cultural institutions and community outreach: What can art therapy do? The Canadian Art Therapy Association. Retrieved from: https://doi.org/10.1080 /08322473.2011.11415549
Coles, A., & Harrison, F. (2017). Tapping into museums for art psychotherapy: An evaluation of a pilot group for young adults. *International Journal of Art Therapy*, 1–10. https://doi.org/10.1080/17454832.2017.1380056
Coles, A., & Jury, H. (2020). *Art therapy in museums and galleries: Reframing practice*. London: Jessica Kingsley.
Elmborg, J. (2011). Libraries as the spaces between us: Recognizing and valuing the third space. *Reference and User Services Quarterly*, *50*, 338–350. https://doi. org/10.5860/rusq.50n4.338
Evans, K., & Dubowski, J. (2001). *Art therapy with children on the autistic spectrum: Beyond words*. London: Jessica Kingsley.
Henry, A., Parker, K., & Legari, S. (2019). (Re)collections: Art therapy training and supervision at the Montreal Museum of Fine Arts ((Re)visiter: formation en art-therapie et supervision au Musée des beaux-arts de Montréal). *Canadian Art Therapy Association Journal*, *32*(1), 45–52. https://doi.org/10.1080/08322473.20 19.1601929
Hyland Moon, C. (2016). Open studio approach to art therapy. In D. E. Gussak & M. L. Rosal (Eds.), *The Wiley Handbook of Art Therapy* (112–121). Wiley Blackwell.
Ioannides, E. (2016). Museums as therapeutic environments and the contribution of art therapy. *Museum International*. https://doi.org/10.1111/muse.12125
Jeffres, L. W., Bracken, C. C., Jian, G., & Casey, M. F. (2009). The impact of third places on community quality of life. *Applied Research in Quality of Life*, *4*(4), 333. https://doi.org/10.1007/s11482-009-9084-8

Kapitan, L., Litell, M., & Torres, A. (2011). Creative art therapy in a community's participatory research and social transformation. *Art Therapy, 28*(2), 64–73. https://doi.org/10.1080/07421656.2011.578238

Legari, S., Lajeunesse, M., & Giroux, L. (2020). The caring museum/Le Musée qui soigne. In H. Jury & A. Coles (Eds.), *Art therapy in museums and galleries: Reframing practice* (1st ed., 157–180). London: Jessica Kingsley.

Leigh-Hunt, N., Bagguley, D., Bash, K., Turner, V., Turnbull, S., Valtorta, N., & Caan, W. (2017). An overview of systematic reviews on the public health consequences of social isolation and loneliness. *Public Health, 152*, 157–171. https://doi.org/https://doi.org/10.1016/j.puhe.2017.07.035

Malchiodi, C. (2007). *Art therapy sourcebook.* New York: McGraw Hill.

Matton, A., & Plante, P. (2014). Le Rôle de L'affichage des Oeuvres en Atelier d'art-Thérapie Chez les Personnes Atteintes du Cancer (Impact of displaying artwork in an open studio workshop offered to people in treatment for cancer). *Canadian Art Therapy Association Journal, 27*(1), 8–13. https://doi.org/10.1080/08322473.2014.11415591

Murzyn-Kupisz, M., & Działek, J. (2015). Libraries and museums as breeding grounds of social capital and creativity: Potential and challenges in the post-socialist context. In S. Warren & P. Jones (Eds.), *Creative economies, creative communities* (145–170). Routledge.

Nolan, E. (2019). Opening art therapy thresholds: Mechanisms that influence change in the community art therapy studio. *Art Therapy, 36*(2), 77–85. https://doi.org/10.1080/07421656.2019.1618177

Ottemiller, D. D., & Awais, Y. J. (2016). A model for art therapists in community-based practice. *Art Therapy, 33*(3), 144–150. https://doi.org/10.1080/07421656.2016.1199245

Parashak, S. T. (1997). The richness that surrounds us: Collaboration of classroom and community for art therapy and art education. *Art Therapy, 14*(4), 241–245. https://doi.org/10.1080/07421656.1987.10759292

Rosenblatt, B. (2014). Museum education and art therapy: Promoting wellness in older adults. *Journal of Museum Education, 39*(3). https://doi.org/10.1080/10598650.2014.11510821

Rowson Love, A., & Szymanski, M. (2017). A third eye or a third space? Systems thinking and rethinking physical museum spaces. In Y. Jung & A. Rowson Love (Eds.), *Systems thinking in museums: Theory and practice* (195–204). London: Rowman & Littlefield.

Simon, N. (2010). *The participatory museum.* Santa Crua, CA: Museum 2.0.

Sloan, L. (2013). *Your brain on art: Art therapy in a museum setting and its potential at the Rubin Museum of Art.* City University of New York. Retrieved from http://academicworks.cuny.edu/cc_etds_theses/398%0AThis

Smallwood, E., Legari, S., & Sheldon, S. (2020). Group art therapy for the psychosocial dimension of epilepsy: A perspective and preliminary mixed-methods study. *Canadian Journal of Counselling and Psychotherapy, 54*(3), 286–323.

Sokoloff, M. (2019). Ouvre-moi: M'acceptes-tu? In E. Corin & L. Blais (Eds.), *Les Impatients: Un art à la marge* (105–115). Montreal: Les Impatients et les éditions Somme toute.

Stiles, G. J., & Mermer-Welly, M. J. (1998). Children having children: Art therapy in a community-based early adolescent pregnancy program. *Art Therapy, 15*(3), 165–176. https://doi.org/10.1080/07421656.1989.10759319

Thaler, L., Drapeau, C.-E., Leclerc, J., Lajeunesse, M., Cottier, D., Kahan, E., . . . Steiger, H. (2017). An adjunctive, museum-based art therapy experience in the treatment of women with severe eating disorders. *The Arts in Psychotherapy, 56*, 1–6. https://doi.org/10.1016/j.aip.2017.08.002

Timm-Bottos, J. (1995). ArtStreet: Joining community through art. *Art Therapy, 12*(3), 184–187. https://doi.org/10.1080/07421656.1995.10759157

Timm-Bottos, J. (2006). Constructing creative community. *Canadian Art Therapy Association Journal, 19*(2), 12–26. https://doi.org/10.1080/08322473.2006.11432285

Timm-Bottos, J. (2011). Endangered threads: Socially committed community art action. *Art Therapy.* https://doi.org/10.1080/07421656.2011.578234

Timm-Bottos, J. (2016). Beyond counseling and psychotherapy, there is a field. I'll meet you there. *Art Therapy.* https://doi.org/10.1080/07421656.2016.1199248

Timm-Bottos, J. (2017). Public practice art therapy: Enabling spaces across North America (La pratique publique de l'art-thérapie: des espaces habilitants partout en Amérique du Nord). *Canadian Art Therapy Association Journal, 30*(2), 94–99. https://doi.org/10.1080/08322473.2017.1385215 LK, https://mcgill.on.worldcat.org/oclc/7251309369

Timm-Bottos, J., & Reilly, R. C. (2014). Learning in third spaces: Community art studio as storefront university classroom. *American Journal of Community Psychology, 55*(1–2), 102–114. https://doi.org/10.1007/s10464-014-9688-5

Treadon, C. B., Rosal, M., & Thompson Wylder, V. D. (2006). Opening the doors of art museums for therapeutic processes. *Arts in Psychotherapy.* https://doi.org/10.1016/j.aip.2006.03.003

11 Museum as Therapeutic Space

Centralizing the Experiences of People of Color

Chloe Hayward

Introduction

In this chapter, I describe my experience with anti-oppression and anti-racist work as an art therapist working in museums. Using my lived experience as a Black woman as the viewpoint for this free-flowing narrative, I explore the intersection of art education and art therapy, and how my theoretical framework informs the creation and holding of therapeutic space within cultural institutions. I identify as a Black woman and speak from the Black experience; however, I want to make space for all People of Color (POC), and that is why you will find these identities represented within the body of this chapter, as I navigate the intersections of Blackness and POC experience. The exploration of the relationship between clinical therapeutic practice and those practices held within community spaces are discussed as means to expand the ways in which community-based therapeutic work is legitimized and consequently made accessible.

Identity, Space, and the Role of Art

There is something about the power of the group that has drawn me to community work over the years, be it the classroom, art therapy groups, or simply a gathering of those who come together for a shared opportunity, as is often the case with museums. Over the years, I have awakened to work which I now understand has allowed me to embark on purposefully and intentionally injecting my voice and my physical presence into spaces that have been traditionally white. This includes the profession of art psychotherapy. My personal background, as someone with a Black father and white mother, raised in a predominantly white town, gave me a plethora of experience as I continue to navigate such spaces.

The work of an art therapist is to create and hold space, and the space I have come to be a part of is working to centralize the experience and voices of people of color. The work is about making space for healing, and it quite often takes place within the space of community. I have witnessed how POC communities come together to give honor and recognition in the collective healing.

DOI: 10.4324/9781003014386-11

The work I am privileged to do in a museum setting is rooted in anti-racism and anti-oppression ideology and provides healing, inclusion, and accessibility through art. Working in museum space – specifically, working for an institution whose mission is anchored in experiences of Black lives and Black culture – I am home. Here there is no need to legitimize my own validity through whiteness. Here, I do not have to worry about being defined by whomever I am in proximity to. I am free to define myself. I am not erased. My identity is not negated based on others' preconceived notions of what identity markers they believe I hold. I do not need to internalize these power dynamics, at best confusing and playing into the protection of white supremacy; at worst making me forget all that I am and all I desire to be in favor of what would best serve the comfort of those around me. For these reasons, I find myself continually drawn to occupy this space and seek to expand, deepen, and enrich the opportunity for others to join me in shaping, creating, and holding this space of creativity. Here, we all find freedom not only to exist, but to shine, and to thrive. To heal. Together. This is why the work of art therapists in museum spaces are so vital. I can testify that my background gives me the experience to hold all of this. To open the space and tend to the emotional recognition and responsibility of those who choose to step into it.

The question is, how do we remain present with all of this: race, identity, comfort, visibility, voice, while centering the POC experience? The answer for me has always been art. It is what helped me dissect my own experiences with identity and race, wrought with emotion. As a therapist I have worked to understand my own relationship to these things so that I may use what I know in recognizing it in others and helping them. In this way, art allows for a richer understanding of self that is cyclical in its ability to heal and expands the ways in which we know ourselves. This in turn helps us to understand and connect to others. The power of art has been proven time and time again as I engage with people of all backgrounds. Through art making and viewing, I am able to facilitate a process that decenters whiteness and centers the Black experience and the experiences of all POC. Art allows the therapist and others working in community settings who hold these spaces to provide reflective distance, to provide a space of safety. We use what we see in front of us to open the space for discussion. We talk about what we see. In the conversation, we reveal the moments we identify with and, more importantly, we evade that in which we do not find a familiarity and comfort. Here lies that opportunity for the art therapist to tap into this discomfort, to make space for revelation that will highlight the ways in which society often favors whiteness and seeks to erase all that is not centered in its supremacist culture. This work allows me to continue to examine with others contemporary context in the critique of societal norms (Gipson, 2017). In this way, I am able to create a space that the traditional educational model alone cannot: by combining my educational pedagogy with psychoanalytic training and framework, and through the lens of my POC lived experience.

The Power of Art

When I became an art therapist, I never thought I would be working in a museum. At the time, I had little understanding of the connections and intersections between art and psychology in museum space. It was something I was unaware of. My career began in education, and I have worked in museums for 20 years. My past experiences in teaching centered predominantly around early childhood demographics. As I worked in a children's museum assisting early childhood lessons, and later in my own preschool classroom, I began to notice much of what I was teaching could be understood through the visual arts. I began incorporating the creative arts process into everything I was doing. Beyond teaching academic goals, I noticed something that (I believe) was much more important: the use of art materials offered students space to address their feelings in ways that words could not. The children and families I served were dealing with a number of financial, emotional, and societal stressors. It seemed absurd to me that we are asking young children to learn and retain information without addressing the emotional part of their self. We were asking parents to show up in ways that were not easy given the inequities they faced. Have you ever tried to memorize or create or think under duress? Not so easy. So why then are we asking children to achieve these amazing academic feats when there may be potentially unaddressed stress or trauma? How are we tending to and growing the social and emotional intelligence of students? Of parents? Of families? Is that not as important? Questions such as these fueled my purpose as I began creating space in my classroom for students to make art in response to their thoughts, their ideas, and their feelings. It became an integrated and integral part of my educational pedagogy.

I witnessed the therapeutic power of art; it was something I was very familiar with in my own life as I addressed my personal journey of self-discovery and emotional growth. As I began to research for any information that could give language to what I was experiencing and witnessing, I came across the field of art therapy. Finally, I had found a discipline that would enable me to incorporate healing through art. As I progressed in my theory and practice, I became more and more critical of the way we, as a clinical community in particular, consider the approach of art therapy. In its tradition, the two schools of art as therapy and art psychotherapy are viewed as interchangeable, given the scope of practice and situation called for. This gives me pause for consideration. Why does it seem we discount the therapeutic value of art and the creative arts process and the healing it holds when it lacks pathology and diagnosis? How might a creative arts process be therapeutic in ways that do not pathologize individuals, while still maintaining "legitimacy" in its results? In what ways is the aspect of "clinical work" connected to the ability of the results and outcomes being considered legitimate? Who owns the right to say whether or not something is legitimate? Where is the space for individuals partaking and leading in the work to engage in ways that are authentic to the community and allow for self-definition? To operate in ways that ignore questions such as these is to participate and advocate for the continuation of a power dynamic rooted in inequity. I believe, much like the ways that some cultural institutions are moving toward a decentering of whiteness so as to create an equitable space, we as art therapists can uplift the community-based path of therapeutic intervention to increase our accessibility. Both museums and art therapy must contend with privilege and the meaning of identity for professional values that have ties to capitalist ideologies that perpetuate inequalities in all areas of human life (Gipson, 2017).

Museums as Therapeutic Space

I keep returning to the notion that, as an art therapist *and* educator working in a museum space, I have witnessed museums as a therapeutic site for healing in community. As I continue to hold space in the intersection between art and psychology, inherently integrative, I am more certain of this with every passing minute. Quite often, it is the magical combination of the artwork being created, viewed, dissected, and discussed that opens the space for healing to take place personally and interpersonally, with self and other, with community and in community. Museums offer a unique opportunity for people to come together and connect, create, and explore conversations around ideas, thoughts, and feelings that aren't always comfortable, but are made accessible through the creative arts process. It's in that reflective distance that we are cracked open just enough to let the light in. Art is a force for self-regulation, for attending to feelings of anxiety surrounding trauma, for seeing and being seen. Museums decenter traditional clinical practice in favor of humanistic, community-based therapeutic approaches providing opportunities for connection and healing. It is why I continue to choose and believe in museums as a space for therapeutic practice. The individuals I hold the privilege to work alongside in an educational, socially engaged arts practice are doing this work as well.

In working as an educator over the past two decades, and most recently as an art therapist in museum settings, I have come to understand the value of being both educator *and* therapist in community space. The combination of the two creates something else, a deeper way of knowing.

My work has become about redefining the relationship between legitimacy and space. My efforts in working in museum space are to promote the legitimacy of nonclinical settings. Art therapy is powerful, and it needs to be given priority in all spaces, broadening its reach and accessibility within a society that deeply needs it. In art therapy, therapeutic spaces do not need to be clinical in order to be effective. In fact, the clinical aspect of this work is what often creates a divide, it is where accessibility is halted in favor of academia. It closes the possibilities of engaging broader communities in the therapeutic value of art and of creative arts processes.

Here is a connection between museum space and therapeutic space to be dissected: quite often these spaces are both white. In my experience, since becoming an art therapist, the profession is in the majority white, and the experiences are often offered through a lens of whiteness. If you are doing this work and it is not rooted in anti-racism and anti-oppression pedagogy, then the lens through which you offer healing can be problematic at best and re-traumatizing at worst. We should all be working in ways that dismantle systems and structures that only view a singular white narrative as definitive of all, regardless of lived experience. It is important for those of us doing this work not only to reflect on our own racialized journey, but to also question our participation in these very systems and structures. Community-based therapeutic art allows for the discovery of disruptive truths and counternarratives of communities often underrepresented and marginalized, *especially* and *particularly* when happening in museum space, which has been historically Eurocentric.

The Role of Racial Identification in Creating Safe Spaces

At the center of all of this is the importance of personal identification to the spaces one occupies. In being able to hold and create space, it is important to understand where you sit within it. How you choose to identify and acknowledge the power and privilege you hold is work which must be done. This is what aids in the creation of safety. Museums are already creating safe spaces to explore identity and the role it plays in understanding oneself and relating to others. In working within a museum whose mission is directly connected to celebrating experiences centered in Blackness, I have witnessed the power of identity and the role it plays in its ability to create safety. As someone who grew up never seeing my image or experience reflected in the spaces I occupied, I have a deeply personal connection to this work. It can be extremely therapeutic to individuals who are able to engage with artworks and artists who look like them.

In witnessing and working within museum spaces to dismantle oppression while elevating the Black experience, I often ask myself: How can museums influence identity formation? Although there have been shifts in more recent times, historically art museums have been institutions that have been white-dominated spaces, implicit in the erasure of the Black experience. In my work over the years, I have come to understand that the role of art therapists in such spaces can include creating conscientious, critically engaged planning that makes room for those whose voices have been silenced in favor of a more palatable narrative, one that protects the fragility of whiteness. I do feel a shift in cultural institutions trying to include more POC voices, and I believe the work that art educators, activists, and therapists are doing in these spaces is creating change. Additionally, and equally as important, as an art therapist I make the effort in my work within cultural institutions to decenter the notion of what is perceived as clinical therapy. I am working to shift the idea of what is clinical and move toward a more holistic, community-based approach that fosters inclusivity and shared authority and supports multiple meaning-making systems. Typical art therapy approaches often ask people to take individual responsibility for their actions, rather than address systems that place POC at risk for an array of consequences stemming from systemic racism (Gipson, 2017). In this way, museums become a space to serve communities as they offer the opportunity through artwork to initiate conversations that address the complexities of race, identity, social justice, and inclusion (Hindley & Edwards, 2017).

The work I do within a museum whose focus is on creating opportunities for the exchange of ideas about art and society, grounded in POC experience, is done through highlighting artists of color and artwork that reflects those experiences. Art provides an opening for POC to come together and see their lives reflected, to see their lives matter. In this way, the museum lives as an anti-oppressive space that disrupts the traditional white-dominated structure of the art institution. It is free to create true inclusion and access, to create community, healing, and change.

Transformation through Community

What might this work look like, based on the theoretical framework and ideologies discussed? What could these therapeutic experiences within a museum space look like? In what ways could the communities they serve benefit? How does this continue to fuel the anti-oppression, anti-racism work of decentering whiteness, shifting what is perceived as clinical, and moving toward a more inclusive, communal space of healing? Individuals dealing with oppressive structures and systems need a safe space for processing their thoughts, feelings, and emotions, some of which reside in the collective unconscious. Museums are a site for the excavation of society's psychological structures and the resulting aftermath groups such as POC experience.

As much of my therapeutic framework is grounded in humanistic theory, I often utilize an approach called open studio. It is the therapeutic lens through which I create all programmatic spaces. This theoretical framework is the link between an art studio and therapy practice, which serves as an alternative to 'clinification' (Allen, 2008). During open studio, the role of an art therapist is to hold the space by being fully present in the creative process, while cultivating a relaxed awareness of or compassionate disinterest in what others are doing. Rather than focus on promoting the therapeutic relationship, the open studio process seeks to promote the relationship between each of us and the artist within, the self, the soul, and the creative expression is witnessed by the community and supports shared engagement. By stepping out of the world of art therapy and its language of "treatment," "therapy," and "diagnosis," we are making an essentially political statement that creativity is more closely aligned to an individual's health than to any disease process. Here, I've witnessed effective spaces for managing racial trauma and healing: no labeling, diagnosing, and categorizing. This is particularly important for POC communities who have a history of stigmatic relationships to mental health and who have had to operate within systems that often further traumatize and oppress. Museums become transformative and empowering spaces to retell stories and personal narratives, allowing the group/individual to change their perception of the trauma. To heal is to transform; in marrying the visual with the verbal, true healing at an integrated level is possible. Rather than simply retelling our stories, we are given the space to change the perception for ourselves and others, to experience rather than avoid. To uplift POC experiences and bring them to the forefront of the conversation. The therapeutic museum space helps expose people (families, adults, teens) to social experiences of the larger society (Smith, 2010) and creates healing within that space for unification through reflection and understanding. The creative arts process aids in the resistance we are so often met with as therapists. In my experience as a Black therapist working within the Black community, I understand how it can be difficult to find treatment that is inclusive of the lived experiences of POC, one that considers the contemporary cultural context. Experiences based in community structures, such as museums, remove stigmatization, pivot how we consider our needs and our lives *in relationship* to those needs, and reduce the limitations to access therapy.

While utilizing an open studio approach means there aren't any particular set goals or outcomes, as is the case with traditional models of education, the creating and holding of such space means people are put at the center of the work and ultimately determine the direction of the conversation and environment. It is the role of the therapist to witness what is brought into the space and offer connective threads through material and verbal interaction. Within the open studio approach, it is the community members themselves who work to share, witness, and support one another. As a result, people are able to experience positive interpersonal connections and relationships, communication, and emotional expression and creativity. Especially in this moment in history, museums need to become spaces for recovery, responding to racial trauma through engagement in a community practice. As finding the language for self-expression isn't always second nature, a therapeutic art experience allows those present to attend to and heal from trauma in community, in safety. Such experiences offer an alternative to traditional pathologizing practices. Within therapeutic spaces, healing occurs as a natural unfolding of the artist's truth is expressed; the more these artists come to know themselves, the more they are able to authentically participate in life and community (Allen, 2008). Here, the museum serves as a safe community space where the lives and experiences of POC are reflected through artwork and the creative arts process, allowing individuals to witness and uplift each other. A museum that values the experiences of Black lives and culture is uniquely positioned to favor a therapeutic arts-based practice as it makes space for the cultural competency necessary to do this work.

Making meaning of our experiences is important, and it is part of the power and the magic of art. Museums that foster an open space where the experiences of POC are reflected in the types of art exhibitions, staff, and visitors are critical in promoting humanity at various levels. Discussions and creative arts processes offered by clinically trained facilitators who are themselves POC or have a deep connection to the POC community through a socially based arts practice are critical. The community-based practice offers art in a way that destigmatizes mental health and encourage the voices of the Black community. It provides a safe space for reflective distance and brings *all* people into the discussion on issues surrounding social justice, gender, race, and identity. Art spaces are inherently therapeutic, and, when held by those whose practices are rooted in anti-oppression and anti-racism, an opening is made not only for an exchange of ideas around art and society, but for a transformation of society itself.

References

Allen, P. B. (2008). Commentary on community-based art studios: Underlying principles. *Art Therapy: Journal of the American Art Therapy Association, 25*(1), 11–12.

Gipson, L. (2017). Challenging neoliberalism and multicultural love in art therapy. *Art Therapy, 34*(3), 112–117. DOI:10.1080/07421656.2017.1353326

Hindley, A. F., & Edwards, J. O. (2017). Early childhood racial identity – The potential powerful role for museum programing. *Journal of Museum Education, 42*(1), 13–21. DOI:10.1080/10598650.2016.1265851

Smith, W. H. (2010). *The impact of racial trauma on African Americans.* African American Men and Boys Advisory Board. Pittsburg, PA: Heinz Endowments. Retrieved from: www.heinz.org/UserFiles/ImpactOfRacialTraumaOnAfricanAmeri cans.pdf

12 Musings on Healing, Museums, and Disability

Marie Clapot

Introduction

I would like to preface this chapter by clarifying my intent. I want to offer some personal musings on how my work as a museum educator concerned with disability and accessibility intersects with wellness and healing outside of an art therapy-based framework. The term 'musings' really best grasps what you are about to read. These musings have occurred over time and keep resurfacing, and so I am grateful to my colleagues, Mitra Reyhani Ghadim and Lauren Daugherty, for ideating this book: *Museum-Based Art Therapy: A Collaborative Effort with Access, Education, and Public Programs*. It has provided me an opportunity to attempt to tie these musings together. I hope they will be thought-provoking and trigger more conversation on the topics of disability and accessibility.

I will start with what my work entails to better understand how access programs at the Metropolitan Museum of Art differ from art therapy-based museum programs. I will explain why this distinction is crucial in fostering access to and equity in cultural participation and in challenging the public perception that disabled people are deficient. This introduction will set the stage to expand on where healing and wellness might appear in access programming and museum experiences more generally. Finally, I will suggest a connection between disability and healing through the interpretation of a work of art by El Greco, *Christ Healing the Blind*.

Art Therapy versus Access Programs

My work as a museum educator is focused on making the Met's collection, exhibitions, buildings, programs, and resources accessible to disabled visitors. This requires the inclusion of accessibility within the broader conversation on diversity, equity, and inclusion. Accessibility is indeed a matter of representation. A space is not truly accessible until it reflects the people it is intended for. Part of our work is to think about how the museum's collection, exhibitions, and interpretation reflect the disability narrative and the ingenuity of disabled artists.

DOI: 10.4324/9781003014386-12

Our goal is to embed accessible and inclusive practices in the overall fabric of the institution through educational programs, museum-wide strategies, and policies. Success lies in a meticulous visitor-centered approach concerned with understanding the multiplicity, complexity, and specificity of the barriers disabled visitors face to cultural participation. Disability is omnipresent. Anyone can become disabled, but not everyone will experience disability the same way. It is a deeply personal experience that is strongly influenced by the cultural, legal, socio-economic, and political systems one lives in. The Met's access programs are designed and tailored to address the ways disability intersects with those systems and identities and stunts the participation of disabled people in the cultural and artistic life of their community. It is also crucial to remember that many individuals live at the nexus of identities. My intent here is to dispel a conflation that I have observed in people. When I share what I do, they often jump to the conclusion that our programs are art therapy programs. No matter how I introduce my work, art programming for disabled visitors becomes associated with art therapy. This unconscious bias feeds the misconstrued belief that arts programming for disabled visitors in museums is systematically tied to art therapy rather than a question of equitable access. It also disregards the myriad of reasons a disabled person visits museums while simultaneously disregarding their agency to choose how to experience museums.

To be clear, museums can choose to offer art therapy-based programs, and there is value in that. Tapping into the potential of museums as places of healing is paramount. But not all access programs in museums are art therapy-based. I cringe at people who tell me I do '*good*' work. I am the victim of my own self-righteousness, impatience, and most likely discomfort with accepting people's graciousness. 'Thank you' would suffice. That being said, as a disabled person and a person who spends time with other disabled folks, I too often experience and witness people's biases and microaggressions. The '*good*' work is not a fight for social justice and equity, it is a "*good cause*" because they perceive us as people in need. They see museums and the arts as the means to repair disabled people's brokenness.

Most disabled visitors come to our programs not because they see themselves as broken or deficient: they opt to participate in an access program because they will be provided with interpretation tools, engagement strategies, and resources that meet their needs should they be blind, have a cognitive impairment, need to sit regularly, or have any other need. Along with finding the necessary support to enjoy their museum experience, participants in access programs also find a community that welcomes and understands them. Families with a member on the autism spectrum will not have to justify or control the stimming of their relative. These behaviors often get stigmatized and cause families to feel 'watched' and ostracized because they don't fit what museum visitor guidelines recommend. Imagine for a minute being that family, constantly on the lookout for the person who is going to make you feel that you need to leave a public place because your relative or friend is disturbing other visitors. Within the space of an access program, this behavior is part of who the person is. Access programs in museums can be healing spaces and offer reprieve from the discrimination and microaggressions disabled people, their friends, and families have to face on regular basis.

Access Programs and Healing

Access programs at the Met are aimed at providing a comfortable space and fostering a sense of community. The programs are structured so that participants enter a space where disability is front and center. While the museum field still has a lot of work to do (us included) towards equal employment for disabled people, we have been striving to hire disabled and Deaf staff, educators, and interns. The point is not mere representation, but to bring disability creativity and ways of thinking and of being in the world to our planning, design, and implementation of strategies and policies. In that sense, it is also crucial to acknowledge the diversity of disability experiences, and that my own experience or that of my colleagues cannot account for the multiplicity of those variations. I strongly believe the presence of our disabled bodies in the space contributes to creating a more accessible space, especially in museums that have been predominantly made by and for nondisabled people.

The programs are not meant *just* for the person with disabilities. Disabled people have social and family lives; they attend programs with friends who might be nondisabled and with family or professional care partners. The programs are inclusive and designed to foster shared experiences. Similarly, a care partner, professional, or a parent should not expect to be there for their relatives, but rather to participate with them. This is an aspect that still surprises people. Years ago, when launching the Met Escapes program for people with dementia and their care partner, I remember two women attending the art-making program for the first time. It became clear that they were mother and daughter. While the mother had been diagnosed with dementia, the disease had serious emotional, psychological, and physical effects on her daughter in the care partner role.

Some of the goals of this program are to reduce the caregiver burden, isolation, and stress by fostering communication and comfort. We aim to utilize the arts to provide opportunities for cognitive, physical, and social stimulation and to improve quality of life for people with dementia and their care partners. As the educator ushered the group into the making component, we set up the supplies in front of each participant, including the care partners. As I approached the daughter, she mentioned to me that she was not going to do the project and was just there for her mother. I acknowledged her and kindly said I would leave the supplies nearby in case she changed her mind. After a few minutes, she tried to get her mother to follow the instructions and quickly became frustrated with her. I came up to her to reiterate my offer for her to participate in the project and to not worry about providing instructions. I assured her our staff was coming to help. She took me up on the offer this time. While I can't remember what was said, I can still clearly picture the daughter getting engrossed in the making activity and engaging in a conversation with her mother about how their creations were turning out. If we had used a device to calculate stress levels, I am almost certain hers would have gone down significantly. Her features loosened, she started smiling, her whole-body language showed more proximity with her mother. In that instance, artmaking as a shared experience clearly alleviated some of the stress in their relationship. Art became an equalizer; they were both focused on creating something. It created an equal footing for them and a place for exchange. In that instance, I could certainly observe some type of healing taking place, but I perceive that healing in its old English meaning of to "make whole."

I think it is worth spending some time looking at etymology here as it gives us a glimpse at some of the differences between art-based therapy museum programs and access programs that do not utilize that framework. The online etymology dictionary (www.etymonline.com) explains that "to heal" comes from the Old English *hælan*, meaning "cure; save; make whole, sound and well" and further says, literally, "to make whole." In the interaction between daughter and mother, no separation existed; namely, the daughter was not viewing her mother as having a disease, nor was she trying to be a caregiver. They were both involved in the activity. In many ways, they were whole. We all experience those moments of wholeness, and I will argue that art is an especially powerful vehicle to bring us closer to those moments.

It is interesting for our purpose to compare this definition with the definition of 'therapy.' The same online etymology dictionary outlines a medical dimension of the practice: "medical treatment of disease," "curing, healing, service done to the sick;" "to cure, treat medically," literally "attend, do service, take care of." That type of healing suggests a problem or something to be treated. Therapy prescribes a tailored intervention and treatment goals. Access programs do not have treatment goals in relation to a specific problem. However, as I mentioned previously, the programs have goals that guide program content and structure.

Healing for All

Earlier, I said that I believed that art is a powerful vehicle to bring us closer to moments of wholeness, of healing. While, in the case of the daughter and her mother at the Met Escapes program, I could observe an example of how being together around art, around a creative activity fostered healing, I think it is important for this upcoming section for you, as a reader, as a museum goer, as an art lover or an observer of beauty, to examine when those experiences might have occurred for you. Can you recall a museum experience that moved you or affected you in some way? Who was there? What were you doing? What happened? What made it memorable?

I would encourage each of you to ask the same questions of family members and friends.

Last summer, I visited the Clyfford Still Museum in Denver, Colorado. I spent a lot of time in the galleries as I was there to prepare for a 4-hour workshop on the role of olfaction in the museum experience and needed to select a couple of works of art from the artist. I knew little about him, his career and practice. So, the process of selecting felt daunting at first. As I slowly made my way through the spacious galleries, taking in decades of practice, I found myself in front of a newly acquired work (*PH-129*, 1949, oil on canvas, San Francisco, CA). This almost 5-by-4-feet large canvas is hung vertically. It is filled with predominantly amorphous jagged forms of light and darker yellows. White outlines some of the spaces created by the irregularity of their lines. In the bottom third of the painting, a grey blue form, probably a foot wide at its largest point, travels through the canvas horizontally, left to right, as if piercing through the yellows. It never reaches the other side of the painting. When travelling upward, my gaze notices more specks of white and a blue emerging here and there and, at the top left, a deep red form seems to want to expand through the yellow.

I stood there for at least 15 minutes, getting closer to examine some details and stepping back to take in the monumental presence of this work of art. Tears came up. They surprised me and pointed out to me that something was happening that I needed to attend to. I stayed with the painting and felt a deep longing to be there, in that world that was unfolding in front of me. My years growing up in a regional park surrounded by the ocean came back to me. Still's jagged blue lines reminded me of the waves crashing against the rocks. Even more than a specific place, specific objects, it was the force, the energy in the planes of yellows, and that burst of red piercing through that brought forth the awesomeness of nature. I felt a sense of place that was not constrained by boundaries or a specific location. It was a world much bigger than I into which I got folded. To me, that was an experience of being whole. Whether you find the words to describe your own experience of feeling whole or not, maybe thinking about it will revive some of the feelings, emotions, or sensations. That is what is important. That is what we can hope for from a trip to a museum. In those moments, there is also a transformation happening. The experience I had changed me. I even surprised myself by remembering it so well from almost a year ago. For me, this speaks to its power.

I believe that the arts are an intrinsic part of the human experience, whether we experience them or make them. I believe we desire to make things beautiful; we seek awesome experiences that remind us we belong to 'something bigger' than ourselves. The arts, as a result or process of artistic practices, are gestures towards expanding on our human experiences of the world. They mimic them and make them grander in the sense that they make the grandiosity of experiences more visible to us.

One of the hallmarks in my practice as a museum educator is to design sensory strategies as a way to connect visitors with works of art and foster a greater understanding. I strongly believe that it is paramount to anchor visitors in their own experience if we want their museum experience to be meaningful. That practice has taught and proved to me that the intellectualization of art can chip away at an experience *with* art. That experience can be based in the somatic or the sensory; it does not require in its duration the involvement of language, but can, and often does, support an articulation of our understanding of a work of art.

Exploring one's own creativity and the creativity of others is an exercise in understanding our own experience, and hopefully an exercise in compassion. Museum experiences are often social. You visit with family, with friends, or you might attend a tour or program. In either case, there is the intimacy of being together with people and of shared experience. We can recognize our differences of opinions and stories or the sharing of similar ones. Those moments are moments of healing and transformation. They open doors to new ways of thinking and to our shared humanity. In that sense, experiencing the arts can heal us by helping us make sense of the chaos of existence.

Challenging Our Understanding of Disability and Healing through Works of Art

A few years back, I led a gallery conversation looking at representations of disabilities in art. The format of the talk was to focus on a single work of art for a full hour. I chose *Christ Healing the Blind* by El Greco (Figure 12.1).

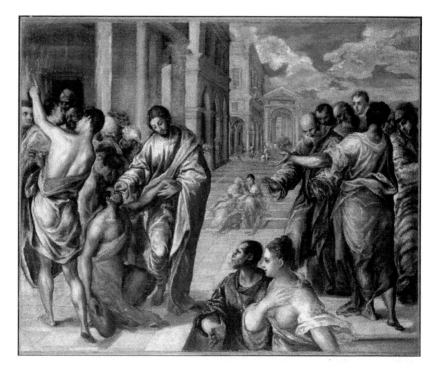

Figure 12.1 Christ Healing the Blind, El Greco, ca. 1570, the Metropolitan Museum of Art

My choice had to do with my own disability, blindness. I am currently legally blind, meaning my field of vision is, at this point in my life, lower than 20 degrees, one of the markers for being medically classified as legally blind. Unless I use my cane, I 'pass' (a term used to define disabled people who, in the binary of ability/disability, appear able-bodied). My father is blind (totally for that matter). Retinitis pigmentosa, a genetic disease that affects the rods and cones in the retina, runs in my family. I grew up surrounded by blindness, fear, guilt, and talk about cures. Since I was 5, my parents have been promising me that, by the time I was older, there would be a cure. I never really cared, maybe because I could play most, if not all, of the sports other kids could. I certainly did not understand the fear around the disease. I am now 39 years old. Research and potential treatments have made leaps, but still no cure. Although I cannot drive anymore and stopped playing some sports for which peripheral vision is crucial, finding a cure is not an objective.

So why is Bartimaeus's story and how El Greco decided to depict him in this event important to me? The painting is housed at the Metropolitan Museum of Art, currently located in Gallery 958 in the Lehman Wing. Two other versions exist that are interesting to compare with the Met's one to appreciate El Greco's enterprise. They can be found in the Gemäldegalerie Alte Meister in Dresden and the Galleria Nazionale di Parma. The oil on canvas, which is about 47 by 57 inches, hangs horizontally above a mantelpiece. The sofa facing it invites you to sit and look up. The painting depicts a scene inspired by the Bible's accounts of St. John and most likely some snippets of St. Matthew's accounts. Three groups of figures are the center of the action. Our attention is drawn to them through the use of a dramatic perspective created by a row of classical buildings to the left of the viewer and blue sky with a few white clouds in the background to the right. In the distance, we can distinguish a carriage lead by horses and other figures going about on the plaza. All are very small in comparison with the three groups in the foreground. The high level of activity is palpable, with gestures guiding our gaze and bright green, blues, and red-colored garments shimmering with light and warm with texture. Closest to the viewer, at the center of the painting, a couple, man and woman, who we can only see from hips to head, are looking up towards Christ and the man kneeling in front of him, Bartimaeus. The couple are his parents. They seem to stand in a pit – a trick to literally set the stage, inherited from the Venetian artist Sebastiano Serlio. From there, our eyes are set on the calm features of the figure of Christ, who seems undisturbed by the commotion around him. He is standing with his right arm softly touching Bartimaeus's face, whose left arm is leaning on Christ's left arm. Christ is accomplishing a miracle before our very own eyes. Next to them, to their right, another man with his back turned to us seems to be pointing towards the sky to the left. He is most likely the second blind man of St Matthew's Gospel, whose vision has already been restored. He is pointing out the light, proving to the group he is talking to that he can see. Huddled to the right of the viewer stand seven figures. Echoing the structure of the group to the left, one of their members has his back turned to us and is talking to the rest of the group. His left arm is outstretched, palm open and facing up. The rest of the figures are all looking where he is pointing. A bearded man is reaching out in the same direction with his right arm, palm facing forward, as if about to stop something. They are the Pharisees, whose attention is turned to the miracle.

The scene captures the miracle being accomplished and other elements from St. John's Gospel, including the Pharisees, who do not believe that the blind man can see and decide to investigate the matter. To their doubt, Christ responded: "for judgment I have come into this world, so that the blind will see and those who see will become blind." To which the Pharisees object: "What? Are we blind too?"

Christ's response: "If you were blind, you would not be guilty of sin; but now that you claim you can see, your guilt remains."

Here, the focus of the healing act is not physical blindness but spiritual blindness. In other words, the Pharisees' lack of faith is their blindness or blind spot. I always wondered about the role of the gestures and touch in El Greco's depiction. As we saw, these gestures support the narrative, but they also bring our attention to touch and the tangible, what is graspable and concrete. In this attempt to capture something intangible, Faith, El Greco builds a visual rhetoric on the senses, their role in perceiving and shaping our ideas of the world, and at once points out their limitation in finding truth.

El Greco paints a topic that is in resurgence at the time because of the Counter-Reformation. The Counter-Reformation sees a reaffirmation of Catholicism after the schism between Catholics and Protestants. After the Council of Trent in 1563, which in essence rejects Protestantism, the Catholic Church reaffirms its basic tenets, which are: Salvation is appropriated by grace through faith and works of that faith. Salvation is gained by the individual's faith alone in trusting Jesus Christ as Lord and Savior. It also emphasizes the use of art to instruct the faithful. El Greco's painting would have been seen by contemporaries as an allegory of the Church of Rome as the embodiment of true faith. It presents the viewer with the questions: What makes us believe? What gives us faith? And it shows God's presence on Earth. Here, 'healing' is about the restoration of wholeness with God. However, the image of the Bartimaeus kneeling at Christ's feet is one that was and is still problematic. Unquestioned, this imagery contributed to and perpetuates a distorted understanding of what the experience of blindness is. Physical blindness is used as a tangible trope to highlight the common lack of faith. While physical blindness is a metaphor for spiritual blindness, the use of the metaphor implies that something needs healing. That there is something wrong with blindness. As a result, the viewer associates the concept of blindness with something wrong. It also can distance the viewer from acknowledging the ways in which they themselves are not experiencing wholeness. Healing for any of us is about recognizing that so often we distance ourselves from what matters most, from what makes us part of the larger fabric of our shared human experience. A deep yearning in all of us to know our place, to know what is means to be utterly ourselves and be open to a world we are totally unprepared for.

Conclusion

This brings me back to an earlier point about the conflation that often occurs in people's minds that access programs must be linked to art therapy. There is nothing inherently wrong with making that connection. It is, however, crucial to acknowledge it might come from a misconception about what the experience of disability is. The person with a disability is often perceived as having a deficiency and lacking something. They cannot go up the stairs, they cannot see, or they cannot speak. The problem sits within the person, not a world (in that case, ableist). That rhetoric built a strong and still persistent separation between an 'us' and 'them' that is making us think that the person needs fixing. It is feeding a belief that disabled people are 'less than.' The truth is that disability creativity is at the source of many innovative museum teaching strategies for exploring works of art and subsequently has enriched everyone's museum experience. While the COVID-19 pandemic is making it clear to all that we all need healing during this trying time, I would suggest that we make healing (whatever shape or form that might take for you) more central to our lives, personal and collective. I strongly believe museums have the responsibility as public institutions to curate healing experiences, in galleries and virtually, for their communities.

13 The Role of Museum Collections in Therapeutic Work

Lauren Daugherty

The use of museum objects in art therapy is an emerging concept that has roots in traditional art therapy practice. In more traditional modes of art therapy, art that clients make is used as a communication tool. Bruce Moon (2017) writes, "Every time a painter fills the brush and moves it across the canvas . . . a proclamation is made to the world: 'I am here, I have something to say, and I am'" (p. 81). For centuries, artists both amateur and professional have been making art to express their beliefs and to process their lived experiences. Art becomes their escape, a coping skill they can use to manage their own emotions and responses. Art therapists in art museums recognize how emotionally charged museum artwork is, and how examining, processing, and responding to works created by other artists can be just as beneficial in treatment as clients creating and exploring their own works of art. "Art that is considered great must communicate at a significant level of meaning" (Wadeson, 2010, p. 4). These objects deemed 'great' are often powerful. They communicate messages that people can only aspire to communicate with words. This thought forms the basis of art therapy. While viewing and connecting with works of art in museum galleries promotes introspection, it is the combination of viewing works of art and reflecting upon them utilizing more traditional methods of art therapy that make the biggest impact. 'Great' art allows people to see something new. Art that clients create allows them to see something new in themselves.

Human Connection with Objects

Humans depend on objects both physically and psychologically (Csikszentmihalyi, 1993). While we physically depend on objects to help us survive on the most basic level, we psychologically depend on objects to help us survive emotionally by allowing them to help stabilize our minds (Csikszentmihalyi, 1993). Museums contribute to this by providing relief from physical tensions and anxiety. Museum artworks have the ability to reflect what is or has been going on in personal relationships and other lived experiences, providing individuals comfort in the face of difficult or stressing times. Objects, including those art objects found in museums, allow individuals to connect with others

DOI: 10.4324/9781003014386-13

through space and time (Silverman, 2010) and to make highly personal connections with works of art, the content within them, and the artists that created them.

Art as Group Member

Donald Kuspit (2010) writes, "The modern artist and her audience are implicitly in a group therapeutic relationship" (p. 1). Artist, artwork, and viewer are all interacting and communicating with one another. In traditional group therapy, the overarching goals are to connect with, learn from, and be supported by others going through similar circumstances. Marian Liebmann (1986) provides a rationale for utilizing group work in a therapeutic context, identifying social learning, mutual support, receiving feedback, trying new roles, and problem solving as advantages of working in groups. But what qualities do museum artworks have that allow an interaction between one singular client and one work of art to replicate that of a group art therapy session? And what makes an experience with art therapeutic?

For an experience with art to be therapeutic, it needs two things: "an artist willing and able to act out her emotional problems and an audience willing and able to empathically reflect on them" (Kuspit, 2010, p. 6). Both of these components are present in museum art therapy programs. Artists willing to act out their emotional problems are present in the museum environment via the works of art on view. Though the artists themselves are not physically present, the works they have created represent who they are and their emotions, values, and beliefs. In museum art therapy, the art therapy client takes on the role of audience member, seeking to connect with artists through their works.

Connections between works of art and audience members exist in group art therapy sessions. Group members present struggles, triumphs, emotions, and other concerns verbally and through images that other group members can connect with and respond to. Group members then reflect upon information presented and offer support, often telling stories about similar experiences or providing words of affirmation and encouragement. This cycle can repeat several times during group sessions when group members present ideas, receive feedback, and apply what they have learned in their daily lives. A similar exchange occurs when clients view works of art in the museum. The works present information to the art therapy client, which the client reflects upon. Through artmaking, the client presents their relationship to the work of art and ideas presented. Clients then take the information they have learned and apply it to their lives outside the museum setting.

Meaning-making

"Viewers have always experienced artworks in relation to themselves" (Cupchik, 2007, p. 18). While museum labels, other interpretive materials, and works of art present information to viewers, museum visitors place more value on the meanings they create when viewing works of art by connecting what they see with their lived experiences (Silverman, 2010). Viewing works of art elicits a variety of emotional and physiological responses in viewers, generally leads viewers to evaluate works they see, and can change lives (Pelowski et al., 2016). When making meaning from objects, internal and external factors build upon each other to create an experience. But how is this done? Neuroscientists studying neuroaesthetics have begun to research how our eyes and brain work together to take in visual information, process it, and attach meaning to the visual world.

Aesthetic Experience Processing Models

"Our emotions color what we notice and how we experience them" (Chatterjee, 2014, p. 25). The things that we notice and emotions connected to them are processed in the brain using parallel processing. We process visual information and attach meaning to it quickly and simultaneously. Chatterjee (2014) outlines the basic structures of the brain and procedures that help us understand what happens in our brains when we take in information and make meaning from what we see. Visual processing of information begins in the retina where we take in visual information. This information quickly travels to the brain and into the occipital lobes, where select areas of this region process shape, movement, and color. These pieces of information merge in the parts of the brain that process faces, places, and objects, ultimately forming visual items we recognize. This process, like most other processes in the brain, happens without our knowledge and occurs rapidly. In museum experiences, this process allows museum visitors to examine a work of art and recognize it as a landscape, portrait, or still life and allows guests to further delineate items within these compositions.

The parts of the brain that allow us to attach meaning and emotion to these visual experiences are housed within the temporal lobes and portions of the limbic brain (Chatterjee, 2014). Meaning-making occurs when portions of these two areas of the brain interact. Personal information relating to our lived experiences is housed in the deepest portions of the temporal lobes, close to the limbic area of the brain where emotions are stored. This limbic area of the brain is closely linked with the autonomic nervous system, which connects our brain and body with emotional experiences.

Leder et al. (2004) break this parallel processing down into five components: perceptual analysis, implicit memory integration, explicit classification, cognitive mastery, and evaluation. In the first component, perceptual analysis, we make simple judgments about a work of art such as if we like or dislike it. Following perceptual analysis, we move into the implicit memory integration component, which consists of processing of which we are not cognizant. Familiarity with the art object and how well the art object fits into our schema of art or specific types of art builds upon our initial impressions, and our brain begins to make an aesthetic judgment about the art object. The next stage of processing, explicit classification, is the point at which individuals can verbalize thoughts about an artwork, typically relating to its content or style. An individual's knowledge about the work of art, artist, or art medium is employed in this component of parallel processing. This information can be presented to viewers via the artwork label, providing context and other art historical or meaningful information about the work. This allows viewers to obtain basic knowledge about the work that contributes to their aesthetic judgment. The final two components, cognitive mastering and evaluation, are closely related, each one informing the activities of the other. The level at which an individual feels they have mastered an understanding of an object changes their final evaluation of it. The simplest way individuals can feel mastery of an object is by relating gathered information from all levels of processing to the self and to their lived experiences, creating a response to the art object that is both cognitive and affective.

Chatterjee (2014) also sees the connection between meaning-making and what we perceive. He proposed a model of aesthetic experience with three levels of information processing: early, intermediate, and late. In the early processing stage, individuals process what they see in very basic elements, including color, shape, and motion. In the intermediate processing stage, a gestalt principle is employed. The brain groups simple elements together to form groups of elements that individuals can make better sense of. Finally, in the late processing stage, individuals can begin to recognize objects and can make meaning from them. They do this by connecting their memories and other associations they have with the content they see.

This parallel processing is also impacted by reflective distance. Reflective distance is typically introduced in art therapy when clients do not have direct contact with an art medium (Lusebrink, 1990). For example, instead of applying paint directly onto a surface using their hands, an art therapist will give clients brushes, sponges, or other tools to paint with. These mediators allow clients to distinguish their own expressions from the sensory input they are receiving from the art medium, placing more emphasis on their visual perception. Although it does take on similar roles in museum art therapy, reflective distance is already present when someone views a work of art, without additional intervention from an art therapist. Because other individuals have created the works of art hanging in museum galleries, art therapy clients do not initially have deep, emotional connections with these works and can easily distinguish their own expressions and reactions from the works of art themselves.

Selecting Museum Artwork for Therapeutic Purposes

Art therapists may consider selecting works of art to utilize in therapeutic programming similarly to how they select art materials to use during traditional art therapy sessions. Individual client or group treatment goals should be considered. Works of art can be selected by art therapists or by clients.

Both methods for selecting artwork can be successful when utilized with the appropriate client or group.

Because each person relates to works of art differently, it can be most informative for art therapists to allow their clients to choose works of art to respond to during museum art therapy sessions. This method of selecting artwork can be particularly impactful in the first art therapy session with a client. When visiting a museum, most visitors gravitate toward something familiar. They utilize their prior knowledge, interests, and experiences to "provide a frame of reference for them to make sense of what the museum contains" (Falk, 2016, p. 97). This allows them to create a sense of security in a new environment. Art therapists can utilize the first artwork a client selects to explore motivations behind the choice of that particular work of art, discussing previous or current experiences that may have played a role in their artwork selection.

Allowing clients to select works of art to view eliminates the role of bias in selecting artwork. Just as each art therapy client or museum visitor brings a unique perspective when viewing artwork, the art therapist connects with works of art based upon their lived experiences. By allowing clients to choose works of art to respond to, the art therapist's past experiences or relationships with specific art objects are not central components of the therapeutic work being done. This ensures that all information presented about artworks relates directly to clients and their experiences with, or interpretations of, artworks.

However, allowing clients to select works of art to view is time-consuming. A large portion of each session in the museum is spent walking around the museum, allowing time for the client to carefully ponder which work(s) of art they would like to discuss and leaving little time for traditional therapeutic interventions to take place. Although it is time-consuming, observing a client interacting in the museum space can provide art therapists with useful information. Clients explore the museum space similarly to the manner in which they explore themselves and their environment (Salom, 2011). The way a client interacts with the museum space can provide therapists with opportunities to discuss boundaries, transitions, permanency, and centrality (Salom, 2011). There are many things therapists can make note of when observing a client in the museum space, including, but not limited to, (1.) if clients are comfortable examining unfamiliar spaces, (2.) if they are respectful of boundaries, (3.) if clients have difficulty transitioning between exhibitions or galleries, and (4.) the process by which they select artworks to discuss.

In larger museums, allowing clients to choose museum artworks for use in art therapy sessions is often an unrealistic goal. The large number of works to choose from can be overwhelming to even the most mentally healthy individuals. If art therapists find that allowing a client to choose works of art to respond to is an important step in meeting treatment goals, they will want to limit the number of artworks their client has to choose from. This can be achieved by the art therapist preselecting a specific gallery or exhibition that most closely relates to the client's treatment goals and that has a wide variety of artworks. Most often, art therapists can achieve this by examining themes present in an exhibition. This strategy can also be useful when working with a smaller group or individuals in museums both big and small. If developing autonomy is an important treatment goal of a small group (six to ten participants), preselecting a gallery or exhibition promotes autonomous selection of artworks. It also allows for a clearly defined space in which the therapist can still observe the group members while paying close attention to how they are interacting within the museum space and with each other. When utilizing this strategy with individual clients in the museum, the therapist can still observe clients in the space while keeping the artwork selection process from taking up too much time during the therapy session.

Allowing clients to have agency over which works of art they would like to view during sessions can also aid in lowering the level of resistance present in museum art therapy sessions. Individuals often approach art therapy cautiously, thinking they have to have artistic talent for art therapy to be effective. Being in the museum environment can exacerbate this and related concerns for clients. Not only do they fear they have to have artistic talent, but they also fear they will not interpret works of art correctly or are not qualified to discuss them at all. These concerns often manifest in resistance to creating artwork or an unwillingness to respond to works of art in the museum. Art therapists can assist in working through this resistance with clients by assuring clients that they can respond to whatever work in the collection they feel most connected to.

If working in a museum where having clients select works of art to view is not attainable, art therapists can choose works of art for their clients to view. This is often the ideal way to integrate viewing works of art with typical art therapy techniques; it provides the art therapist with an opportunity to choose works of art that directly correlate to treatment goals and provides more time during sessions for traditional therapeutic work to occur. Works of art can often be connected to treatment goals explicitly through themes or subject matter. Themes present in works of art are endless and do not have to come from museum labels or other interpretive materials used in exhibitions. These themes should focus on the client(s) and should be less about art historical information or the artists' interpretations of artworks. An art therapist might choose to relate a highly complex abstract painting with what the feeling of anxiety might look like, or could choose to connect a treatment goal of working through abuse and neglect by discussing family relationships between the individuals found in a family portrait. Art historical information, information about the artist, or details of the process the artist used to create the work of art should only be discussed if brought up organically by the client or if mentioning these facts contributes to the connection between the work of art and treatment goals.

By selecting works of art to view in art therapy sessions, the art therapist is able to provide structure. Structured art therapy sessions can be beneficial for clients with treatment goals related to anxiety, Alzheimer's disease and dementia, intellectual and developmental disabilities, as well as children and teens working on emotion regulation. Having these clients choose artwork to view and respond to in art therapy sessions could be emotionally overwhelming, creating an unnecessary stressor in the therapeutic space, which could impact the amount of progress individuals are able to make in museum art therapy programming. By taking control of the art selection process at first, the art therapist provides a space in which his/her clients can be most successful, eventually working up to clients selecting their own works of art to respond to, if it is determined that this will help them reach their goals.

Museum-based Art Therapy: A Space for Personal Growth and Reflection, an Art Therapy Experience at the Sidney and Lois Eskenazi Museum of Art

In collaboration with Indiana University Lifelong Learning, I led an art therapy group for adults age 18 and older. Museum Art Therapy: A Space for Personal Growth and Reflection provided participants with an opportunity to relate our museum's collection to their lived experiences and witness how the museum can contribute to personal healing and well-being. In three 90-minute sessions, the group participated in gallery-based experiences, artmaking for reflection, and discussions about their overall experience in the museum spaces. Each of the three sessions and their content are outlined below.

Session 1

The group began with an introduction to art therapy and an art-making experience in the museum's artmaking studio. I explained art therapy as a profession, how it is utilized at the museum, and what types of experiences they could expect in the galleries and in the artmaking studio.

Because there was not enough time for the group to participate in both in-gallery and artmaking experiences, I selected an artmaking exercise for the group to complete that would serve multiple purposes: (1.) introduce the group to the overall content of the three sessions; (2.) allow the group a chance to explore the artmaking studio and materials, ultimately gaining comfort in the space; and (3.) begin to establish a group connection through sharing of their artwork. I asked the group to take a moment to imagine what their souls looked like, really examining their inner selves and beginning to think about how they might represent that visually. All art materials in the artmaking studio were made available for this directive, and participants were given 45 minutes to create artwork. Responses ranged in media from collage and other drawn images to 3D sculptures made from air dry clay, papier-mâché boxes, string, and chenille sticks. Some participants chose to make material choices that allowed them to portray their versions of their souls or internal self in specific colors, while some modeled their souls to be specific shapes or forms. A range of materials was offered for this directive to allow for many types of visual representations and to allow each group member to select materials they were comfortable with using. The directive itself was very abstract and required the participants to be somewhat vulnerable, making comfort level with materials important during this session. Many participants had previous experience with art materials beyond the traditional high school level, and I was confident they could select art materials they would be successful using.

Session 2

Utilizing a participant-led method for selecting artwork, I asked the group to explore the museum's gallery and identify something that was missing in their lives, or something they wish they could change about their current lived experience. I asked them to think back to the works of art they created during the first session and identify an area of their 'soul' that was not complete. We then entered the galleries, where participants had about 45 minutes to explore the collection and choose an image. Participant 1 selected the painting *Valley of Mexico from the Tepeyac* (Figure 13.1) to discuss with the group. This painting depicts the valley of Mexico City with Lake Texcoco in the background. While Participant 1 was describing the content of the image to the group, he began to discuss his personal connection to this image. Born in Mexico, Participant 1 grew up not far from the location depicted in the painting and stated the image reminded him of the family he still had in Mexico. He stated he did not speak

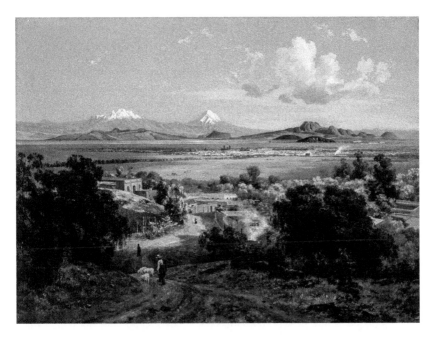

Figure 13.1 Valley of Mexico from the Tepeyac, José María Velasco, 1895, Eskenazi
Museum of Art, Indiana University, 75.117.1

with them as much as he would like to, and that "viewing this painting was a nice reminder of how important maintaining connections with loved ones is, even if they be only spiritual connections with happy memories, and where it might not be possible to maintain a long-distance physical connection."

Participant 2 selected Alfred Leslie's work *Portrait of Lisa Bigelow* and discussed her relationship with the figure in the portrait with the group. The painting is a larger-than-life-size image of a woman in black, white, and gray tones. The participant stated,

> Lisa in the painting seems to be at a point that I was when I was her age – she seems to be perhaps late twenties, or maybe even thirties. She seems experienced beyond her years. Her very short hair would indicate a lack of femininity. Her eyes are huge and very sad, her expression is questioning. Her stance in the picture is perhaps inviting you in to touch her, or looking for company. She seems peaceful, yet melancholy. She is protecting her misery, or dealing with some pain and ready to move on. She also seems like a large girl and I relate to that. When I was that age, I had just emerged from about a decade of extreme psychological distress starting in my late teens. I felt hopeless and colorless, hence the gray tones, unsmiling face, and hesitant stance. At the same time, the largeness of the picture indicates to me that Lisa B. has the power to battle her inner demons, whatever they are . . . [Leslie's] depiction of her is very honest and I relate to that.

Session 3

In our third and final session, I asked the group to explore the museum's galleries and find a symbol of strength. I challenged participants to think back to the two previous sessions and utilize this session as an opportunity to think and reflect upon what aspect of themselves could provide them strength to repair the missing part of their souls they identified in Session 2. Participant 3 identified *Pair of Earrings* (Figure 13.2), attributed to the Maasai Peoples of Kenya, as an object she identified with.

The earrings are rather large and are made from small, brightly colored beads strung together in an intricate pattern. The participant recalled jewelry always being a way for her to express herself and her identity. To her, jewelry is a symbol of female strength. She also connected the imperfections in the earrings to Western culture's relationship to perfection and her own artmaking practice, stating,

> In Western culture, we often celebrate balance and perfectionism, but in their culture, imbalance and differentiation was considered beautiful. I connected this to my own approach to art-making and the way I view beauty. It felt very validating to discover a perspective that was similar to my own.

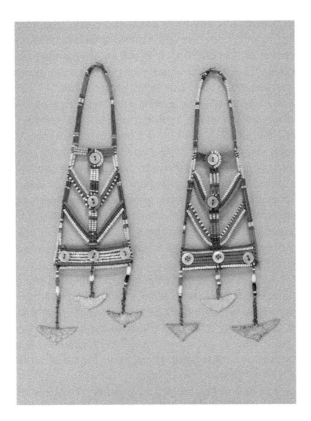

Figure 13.2 Pair of Earrings, Maasai Culture, Kenya, 1930, Eskenazi Museum of Art
Indiana University, 2009.7

Secondary Meaning-making

Museum-based art therapists have their own personal connections to works
of art. Our lived experiences impact what work we find meaning in and how
we emotionally connect with those works. However, there is another form of
meaning-making, one that does not draw from personal lived experiences.
This type of meaning-making is impacted most by our clients' lived experiences. As any type of therapist will tell you, the stories of our clients lie
within us. We are the holders of happy memories and traumatic events that
are not our own.

Portrait of Lisa Bigelow

In the art therapy group mentioned previously, one participant found a deep
connection with *Portrait of Lisa Bigelow* by Alfred Leslie. Just to put the
image in your mind's eye again, the portrait is a larger-than-life-size rendition

of a woman completed only in tones of gray. She has short hair, almost giving her a manlike appearance. She has a blank expression, and her arms hang at her sides. She is clothed in a sleeveless dress. A favorite work of mine in the Eskenazi Museum of Art collection, it struck me the moment I saw it. To me, Lisa looks strong. This strength is something I have seen in very few living beings, but was something that I saw in my grandmother.

When I was 15 years old, my grandmother was diagnosed with ovarian cancer, a disease that eventually took her life. My grandmother was strong, not physically, but mentally – where I think strength matters most. I knew she was in pain, that she had to be feeling isolated, and that she wished cancer had never become a part of her life. She never mentioned any of that. She always smiled when my family came to visit her in the hospital. She was always concerned with how my grandfather was doing and wanted to hear about my sister and my latest volleyball game. We didn't talk about her cancer, but you could see all of her thoughts about it in her eyes. Like Lisa, she was strong, yet anyone who saw her would tell you there was a lot going on under the surface.

Each time I walk by this work in the gallery, I think of my grandmother. Yes, I think about her cancer, but I think about much more than that. I think about the quilt I have at home that she made me out of my dad's old shirts. I think about the trips my sister and I took to the hardware store with both her and my grandfather to get snow cones. I think about the countless times we went over to her house to swim in the pool. I think about the wonderful life she lived.

But now, when I look at *Portrait of Lisa Bigelow*, after I have thought about my grandmother, I think about Participant 3 and her connection to Lisa. I think back to that art therapy group and smile, knowing just how powerful works of art can be in connecting us with our lives and the lives of others – past, present, and future.

Summary

Museum collections can play important roles in art therapy programs. As art therapy programs in art museums gain popularity, it is important that art therapists increase their understanding of how to utilize museum artworks in therapeutic work. Works of art are emotionally charged. Art therapy clients and art therapists can interact with and gain meaning from these works of art just as they would another group member in a more traditional art therapy experience. Just as artmaking is personal and reflects lived experiences of the individual engaging in the creative act, viewing works of art has the same capability. Looking at art can reflect past and current experiences and realities. Capitalizing on the power works of art have to serve as catalysts for discussion and therapeutic work is integral in museum art therapy and can provide additional points of entry for clients who are hesitant to engage in their own artmaking.

References

Chatterjee, A. (2014). *The aesthetic brain: How we evolved to desire beauty and enjoy art*. New York City, NY: Oxford University Press.

Csikszentmihalyi, M. (1993). Why we need things. In S. Lubar & D. Kingery (Eds.), *History from things: Essays on material culture* (20–29). Washington and London: Smithsonian Institution Press.

Cupchik, G. C. (2007). A critical reflection on Arnheim's gestalt theory of aesthetics. *Psychology of Aesthetics, Creativity, and the Arts, 1*(1), 16–24.

Falk, J. H. (2016). *Identity and the museum visitor experience*. New York City, NY: Routledge.

Kuspit, D. (2010). *Psychodrama: Modern art as group therapy*. London: Ziggurat Books.

Leder, H., Belke, B., Oeberst, A., & Augustin, D. (2004). A model of aesthetic appreciation and aesthetic judgements. *British Journal of Psychology, 95*, 489–508.

Liebmann, M. (1986). *Art therapy for groups: A handbook of themes, games, and exercises*. Newton, MA: Brookline Books.

Lusebrink, V. B. (1990). *Imagery and visual expression in therapy*. New York City, NY: Plenum Press.

Moon, B. L. (2017) *Introduction to art therapy: Faith in the product* (3rd ed.). Springfield, IL: Charles C. Thomas.

Pelowski, M., Markey, P., Lauring, J. O., & Leder, H. (2016). Visualizing the impact of art: An update and comparison of current psychological models of art experience. *Frontiers in Human Neuroscience, 10*, 1–21.

Salom, A. (2011). Reinventing the setting: Art therapy in art museums. *The Arts in Psychotherapy, 38*, 81–85.

Silverman, L. H. (2010). *The social work of museums*. New York City, NY: Routledge

Wadeson, H. (2010). *Art psychotherapy* (2nd ed.). Hoboken, NJ: John Wiley.

14 Practical Methods and Strategies

Lauren Daugherty and
Mitra Reyhani Ghadim

Introduction

In this chapter, we aim to offer practical tools and strategies that can be flexibly utilized within museum-based programs. We pair select strategies with examples featuring their use and implementation. Methods have been selected from findings from successful programs over the years, as well as cumulative action research and experimentation through numerous museum art therapy projects. The evolution of these museum art therapy best practices was made possible by years of passionate, creative, and dedicated collaboration and contributions made by museum art therapists and art therapy interns, museum educators, and teaching artists.

Practical Methods and Strategies

The intersection of personal and shared interests with gallery-based activities produces new, flexible, creative, and meaningful entry points for the access of audiences. The experience of individuals interacting with museums and their collections' objects, including those contents' intrinsic, physical, and material properties, generates sensory, emotional, and cognitive associations, memories, and projections (Froggett, Farrier, & Poursanidou, 2011). The work of the museum professional is to create situations and entry points for these interactions. The engagement and interactive experience of individuals can involve a process where museum objects function as symbols of identity, relationships, nature, society, and religions (Pearce, 1995). Below is an outline of four categories that museum art therapists and other wellness professionals can use when developing activities for engagement with museum artworks. These categories were developed collaboratively by one of the authors of this chapter in her position as manager of the art therapy program at the Queens Museum, the program's full-time coordinator, Rachel Shipps, and art therapist Jennifer Candiano (2018) and describe some findings from the PAVE guide, a program that was briefly described earlier in Chapter 4 of this book. The categories are as follows:

- Verbal exchange
- Kinetic experiences and activities

DOI: 10.4324/9781003014386-14

- Connecting by making in the galleries
- Multisensory experiences

Works of art from the Eskenazi Museum of Art at Indiana University Bloomington accompany these categories, along with our own responses as examples. We have provided responses or ideas on how we might use these images in a therapeutic way or in a wellness program. It is important to note that the responses we give are just examples. Every client or participant will respond to works of art differently.

Verbal Exchange

Verbal communications in the galleries are an excellent way of sharing personal connections, evoking imaginative and narrative qualities of museum objects, and sharing background information. Consider, as you plan verbal exchanges, that some participants may use other language styles than those on museum labels. A *verbal exchange inquiry* in a museum or gallery can involve step-by-step processes.

1. Begin with a theme or objective
2. Use questions that are open-ended and encourage observation. You may begin by asking, "What do you notice?" "What do you see?" You could also utilize a thinking routine such as See, Think, Wonder, created by Project Zero of the Harvard Graduate School of Education (Project Zero, 2016)
3. Make sure to give time for a variety of responses and ask if people have anything to add
4. Ask viewers to use their observations as evidence for any conclusions they draw
5. Inquiry for engagement and meaning making begins with observation and open-ended questions. As facilitators, we do not want to give yes/no, true/false answers to questions. Instead, we can compare, contrast, and connect visitors' perspectives and questions and add in facts as topics arise
6. Allow the viewer to make immediate personal connections by using questions such as "What memories and feelings are associated with this object or the displayed art?"
7. Based on the object or artwork, you can be very specific or very general

Examine *The House on the Moor* (Figure 14.1) while thinking about the following forms of verbal exchange. Think about how your responses differ or match the ones we have included and begin to think about a work of art you might use to engage an art therapy client or participant in a form of verbal exchange.

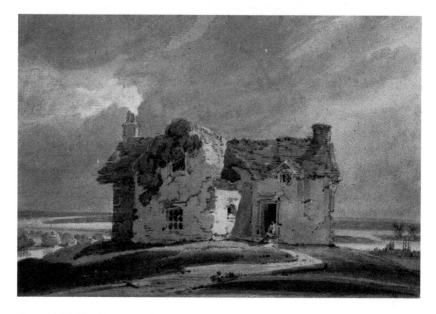

Figure 14.1 The House on the Moor, Thomas Girtin, 1801–02, Eskenazi Museum of Art, Indiana University, 68.129

Visual Thinking Strategies

Using art looking and artmaking to spark conversation forms the essence of museum-based art therapy. *Visual thinking strategies* (VTS) is another arts-based inquiry method. Developed by Abigail Housen and Philip Yenawine, VTS is a teaching strategy which encourages communication and visual literacy (Housen & Yenawine, 2020). When VTS is utilized as a method that aligns well with art therapy, the artworks and/or art concepts are not the center of attention for their art historical significance or for the craftsmanship and skill of the artist, but for their potential to initiate conversation and reflexivity, as well as promote participatory learning. As in verbal exchange in art therapy, VTS allows each person to feel that their observations and thoughts are valued, as they collectively build upon each person's individual perspective.

Three questions frame the discussion:

- What's going on in this picture (artwork)?
- What do you see that makes you say that?
- What more can we find?

As you hear from each participant, rephrase what they have said, recognizing their own words and introducing related ways of speaking about the same topics. Point to the work of art or object to indicate their specific focus. As people agree or contradict each other, note this without judgment. Participants are finding out information and creating meanings individually and/or together as a group. For this exercise, we will assume our clients are a group of veterans experiencing loss of sense of purpose, hopelessness, and anxiety about their transition from active duty to civilian life. The following is an example exchange that could occur when looking at this image;

Facilitator:	What's going on in this image?
Participant 1 (Carlos):	There is a lonely man sitting in the doorway of an abandoned house.
Facilitator:	Carlos sees a man sitting in the door of an old house and thinks the man is lonely. What do you see that makes you say that, Carlos?
Carlos:	The house looks really old, and there isn't anything else around it. The colors are very gloomy, and there are no other people in this image. The colors make me feel the man is lonely.
Facilitator:	Carlos thinks how the house looks makes it appear abandoned and that the gloomy colors the artist used give him the feeling the man is lonely. What more can we find?
Participant 2 (Allison):	I see smoke coming from the chimney.
Facilitator:	Allison sees smoke coming from the chimney. What do you see that makes you say that, Allison?
Allison:	The artist has used a different color to illustrate the smoke. It makes me think the man isn't alone. There might be someone else inside.
Facilitator:	Allison thinks the different color the artist used to illustrate smoke shows that there might be another person inside the house.

This exchange would continue for as long as time permits. Encourage everyone to participate and ask for a response from group members who tend to be quiet, sometimes extending an invitation to share their opinion. If an art therapist is facilitating, they may make mental notes about things group members brought up that could be used in the formation of an art directive or further discussion and exploration. With this example group, an art therapist may find it would be helpful for the group to create their own artwork about that feeling of loneliness. What does it feel like inside their body? What supports do they have in place to help them combat those feelings when they arise? An art therapist may also use the image of the house as a metaphor for the self and ask participants to draw what their 'Self house' looks like. The therapist could follow up with additional questions. How do people get in your Self house? Are there certain people you would let in and certain people you would not? What is it like to live in this house?

Place Yourself in an Artwork

Imagining oneself in the artwork can take very different forms and bring sensory perspectives to an experience with an art object. You can ask a variety of questions to help participants imagine themselves in an artwork. How would it *feel* to be in this painting? How would it smell? What emotions would you be *feeling*? What sounds would you hear? Where would you go first in this image? Where would you go in this image to feel safe? For this exercise, let's imagine the client is a young child in the foster care system coping with post-traumatic stress disorder symptoms. If a facilitator were to ask this child where they would go first in the painting, the child might respond with "I would go to the water," or, if a facilitator asked this child what emotions they would be feeling if they were in this painting, they may respond with "Sad. I would be alone."

Improvisation Techniques in Art Therapy

Improvisation is a well-known form of entertainment first developed in the theater, based on non-rehearsed interactions. During the past decade, improvisation has grown in popularity as a method for learning and engagement. Because improv depends on the group providing support for every answer, participants also grow in confidence and feel more connected to others (Flanagan, 2015), which can have significant meaning for building rapport with participants in art therapy. For the exercises below, imagine you are working with a group of adolescents working on building self-confidence and self-esteem.

Yes, And

The first person notices something in the artwork and states what they see. The next person says "*yes*" and repeats exactly what the person before said, then adds, "*and*" something they see.

Alex: I see a house.
Lindsey: Yes, you see a house, and I see water.
Alicia: Yes, you see water, and I see sky.

I Think, I Wonder

Alicia: I think that house looks a bit creepy.
Alex: Yes, you think that house looks a bit creepy. I wonder if the man is scared to go inside.

Sell the Story

Look at a work of art and have participants work in pairs or individually to come up with a "story" they see in the artwork. Have the group present the story to one another as "fact." For an art therapy approach, the participants create a story that holds metaphors or meanings that may be easier to express through a fictional narrative. Group members are prompted by these questions to provide evidence for stories and inferences, and all entry points to art viewing are validated. As people make observations, facilitators point and indicate the area they are referring to and rephrase the question, reaffirming observations and making new meanings visible. Think back to that group of veterans we mentioned earlier. Carlos creates a story and shares with the group. From here, an art therapist may think about ways to incorporate art-making into the process. Could participants illustrate a portion of the story not illustrated by the work of art? Can they create an alternate ending to the story if desired?

Free Word Association

In a small group format, look at a work of art and generate one word per person. Choose one word to start with, say that word (example: arrow), and then ask for the "first word that comes to your mind." The group should keep associating words with the first word that comes to their mind. After a list is generated, look back at the artwork together. This technique allows for the group's collaborative meaning constructions that support both the group formation and intersubjective exchange. You can also record the list and play it back or write everything down and review together. See how observations change. Using the adolescent group as a model, a verbal exchange might be: House (first word). Home. Mom. Rules. Freedom. And so on. After a verbal exchange like this, an art therapist could ask the group to explore those concepts of rules and freedom in their own artwork.

Kinetic Experiences and Activities

A physical activity that allows the individual to develop a bodily sense and "feel" for the concept that is being offered visually or that is being described offers a different understanding that is often more compelling than a concept that remains an abstract thinking activity. Physically acting out knowledge to be learned or problems to be solved makes the conceptual metaphors employed by our brains a literal reality (Murphy, 2014). Examine *Tweezers* (Figure 14.2) as you discover some examples of physical/movement activities that can be used in museums and galleries. Can you imagine a group of children, adolescents, or adults completing these activities with this work of art?

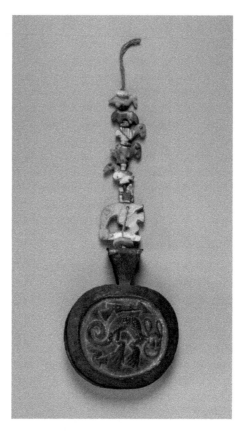

Figure 14.2 Tweezers, Chimú Culture, Peru, 1100–1300, Eskenazi Museum of Art, Indiana University, 72.21.4

Mimicking Art Objects

- Mimic the posture of an artwork: examine the posture of the figure, replicate how that figure is standing
- Mimic the emotion of the artwork: identify an emotion or feeling and use body and facial expression to act it out or share it
- Use motion to imitate shapes and lines: brushstrokes, forms, lines, and borders are all evidence of a maker's process and can be reenacted with the body. Pace and speed can also help access the technique and feeling behind an art object. In a group, find a line or a shape in a work of art. Pose like it, one person at a time. Continue to add until everyone is part of the pose. You can add movement and sound. For example, if a group is posing like a line found in one of the animal figures in *Tweezers*, encourage them to also mimic the sound that line or animal might make

Connecting by Making in the Galleries

How do we use galleries for engagement, learning, and enrichment? Experiential learning, or learning by doing in the gallery, is real, exciting, and a meaningful, active way of learning for children with their parents or caregivers as partners. Using the image of *Nissaka Station* (Figure 14.3) as inspiration, discover examples of hands-on activities for use in museum galleries.

Sketching/ Drawing

Pencils, paper, and cardboard can be offered for quick sketches in the galleries. Drawing can be an artistic, perceptive, and imaginative response to the exhibit, the art, or the experience. In addition to sketching from observation, participants may add words or create an imaginary environment for the art object. In *Nissaka Station*, it appears as though a group of individuals are walking up the

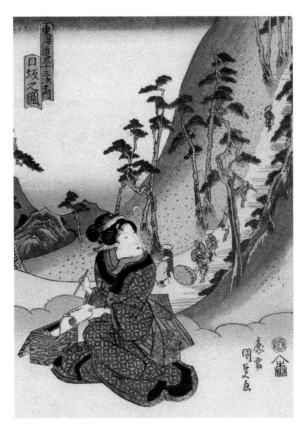

Figure 14.3 Nissaka Station, Utagawa Kunisada, 1838–42, Eskenazi Museum of Art Indiana University, 2012.80

path on the hill or mountain. A facilitator could ask participants to draw what they might find at the top of the hill.

Writing

Constructing a story, rehearsing personal memories or narrative, creating an interior monologue based on the subject of an artwork or a poetic response are all options for written interactions. Participants can develop and focus their observations with the aid of written rehearsal. There appears to be a woman writing something in *Nissaka Station*. A facilitator might ask the group to write what they think she is writing down on her scroll, ask the group to create a written narrative of what the group of people in the background are saying to each other, or ask each group member to write a story about what is happening in the image.

Make Stations

Using museum curator-approved artmaking materials, the activities offered in the gallery are designed as inspired by the specific exhibit, art piece, or theme that is in close proximity. Tape, paper, pencils, kraft paper, masking tape, aluminum foil, chenille sticks, and art straws are examples of materials that could be used in museum galleries. Make sure to always check with each institution to see what materials are allowed in its galleries before creating a make station. A make station in conjunction with *Nissaka Station* could involve various 3D materials approved for gallery use, so that museum guests could create their own versions of some of the natural elements in the work. A make station could also use those same 3D materials and some drawing materials to encourage guests to create their own attire like the clothes of the woman in the work of art.

Multisensory Experiences

The following sample tools promote engagement while also allowing for the visitor to be self-directed in the galleries. The tools can attract children and family members without intimidation and without requiring a verbal prompt and/ or by providing visual and tactile appeal. Tools can take the form of interactive objects designed to be carried into the galleries, or shared points of contact between gallery staff and visitors. Special attention must be given to the cleaning of tactile objects and use of gloves for hygienic safety. Examine *Le Bassin d'Argenteuil* (*The Port of Argenteuil*) in Figure 14.4 and imagine what types of multisensory experiences you might create for this and other works of art.

Interactive Boards

Written or verbal prompts inspire visitors to respond to an exhibit by leaving questions, personal recollections, or ideas on a public display board in the

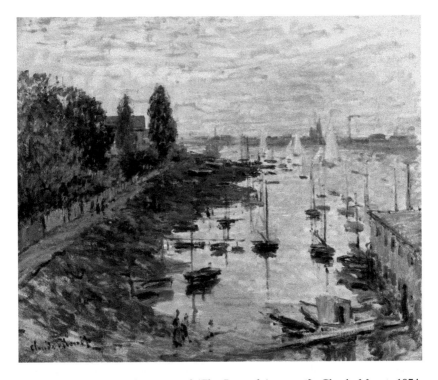

Figure 14.4 Le Bassin d'Argenteuil (The Port of Argenteuil), Claude Monet, 1874, Eskenazi Museum of Art, Indiana University, 76.15

galleries. With each experience, we ask ourselves how we can make prompts more inclusive, considering language use and multiple means of representation. Boards may be designed to be replaced at the end of each day. Interactive boards can also be digital when possible.

Tactiles

Focusing on a texture, technique, material or form, tactile models are built of exhibit objects or objects inspiring an exhibition. They may be created by hand or in some cases purchased from model-making companies or companies that use 3D printers. Visitors interacting with tactiles may acquire a new sense of scale, shape, medium, or texture. Tactile models are excellent tools for engagement for individuals with varying speech, sight, hearing, or cognitive levels. With the consideration of safety after the worldwide experience of the pandemic, ongoing cleaning and use of gloves must be made available to ensure hygienic protection. A tactile model of *Le Bassin d'Argenteuil (The Port of Argenteuil)* could emphasize the brushstrokes in the work. Other tactile boards or experiences with this work of art could include materials mimicking the textures of some of the natural elements such as water, sand, and grass, or could mimic textures found on the sails of the boats in the port.

Audio Interactives

Audio interactives may be used not only to diversify the methods of interpretation provided by the museum, but also to support the idea that there is more than one way to view, experience, and relate to artworks. Anything from multilingual guides to recorded personal impressions of artworks may serve a range of visitors who prefer sound as an interpretive mode and bring new voices into the museum. Such intersections of interpretation and education provide opportunities for collaborative work between curatorial and education staff. An audio interactive for *Le Bassin d'Argenteuil* (*The Port of Argenteuil*) could include sounds of water, nature, or voices like those you would hear in the port, but could also include audio about the work of art, the artist, or the time period it was created and audio descriptions of the work of art for individuals who are blind or have low vision.

Conclusion

There are many ways art therapists and other wellness professionals can use works of art to begin discussions. We have highlighted some methods of engaging with works of art in this chapter that you can replicate using works of art in any museum or gallery. When selecting a method of engagement, always be sure to select a method that focuses on a group's or individual's strengths and that meets the needs and purpose of the group. For example, a group of individuals with autism or other sensory processing disorders may benefit more from a tactile experience that engages more of their senses and offers sensory support, as opposed to strictly verbal processing of a work of art. A group of children with ADHD may benefit from something kinetic in the galleries where they can move their bodies. No matter the method of engagement you choose for your audience, works of art are rich with information that can lead participants to discover more about the artworks, themselves, and the world around them. However, these works of art are just the beginning of the discussion; see what more information you and your participants can learn by engaging in artmaking alongside these types of exchanges in a museum or gallery.

References

Candiano, J., Dejkameh, M., & Shipps, R. (2018). Paving new ways of exploration in cultural institutions. A gallery guide for inclusive arts-based engagement in cultural institutions. Queens Museum

Flanagan, L. (2015). How improv can open up the mind to learning in the classroom and beyond. Retrieved from: www.kqed.org/mindshift/39108/how-imrov-can-open-up-the-mind-to-learning-in-the-classroom-and-beyond

Froggett, L., Farrier, A., and Poursanidou, K. (2011). Who cares? Museums, health and wellbeing: A study of Renaissance North West Programme. University of Central Lancashire. Retrieved from: https://eresearch.qmu.ac.uk/bitstream/handle/20.500. 12289/4726/4726.pdf?sequence=1&isAllowed=y (accessed December 6, 2020).

Housen, A. & Yenawine, P. (2021). Visual thinking strategies. Retrieved from: vtshome.org

Murphy, P. A. (2014). Let's move! How body movements drive learning through technology. Retrieved from: www.kqed.org/mindshift/36843/lets-move-how-body-movements-drive-learning-through-technology

Pearce, S. M. (1995). *On collecting: An investigation into collecting in the European tradition.* Routledge.

Project Zero. (2016). See, think, wonder. Retrieved from: https://pz.harvard.edu/resources/see-think-wonder

Index

Note: Locators in *italic* indicate figures, in **bold** tables.

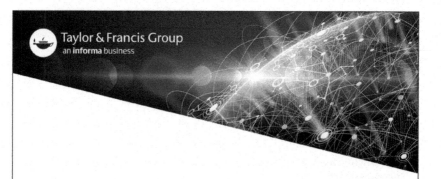

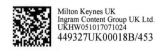
Milton Keynes UK
Ingram Content Group UK Ltd.
UKHW051017071024
449327UK00018B/453